Taste of Goldie

Welcome to Taste of Goldie, Where Every Dish Tells a Story and Every Flavor is a Journey. Here, We Celebrate the Art of Cooking by Bringing Together the Freshest Ingredients, Time-honored Recipes, and a Sprinkle of Love. Our Kitchen is a Vibrant Tapestry of Cultures, Flavors, and Culinary Traditions, Where We Invite You to Explore the Magic of Food. Whether You're a Seasoned Chef or a Curious Novice, Taste of Goldie is Your Gateway to Discovering the Joy of Cooking. Join Us as We Embark on a Delightful Adventure, Transforming Simple Ingredients Into Extraordinary Meals That Will Tantalize Your Taste Buds and Warm Your Heart. Let's Create Something Beautiful Together!

With love
Kang Aplow

Introduction

Welcome to "Goldie's Gourmet Adventures," Where Every Recipe is a Cherished Tale Waiting to Be Told! Nestled Within These Pages Are Not Just Ingredients and Instructions, but a Vibrant Tapestry of Memories, Laughter, and Love. Picture This – the Aroma of Freshly Baked Bread Wafting Through the Air, the Sizzle of Spices Dancing in a Hot Pan, and the Warmth of Shared Meals That Linger Long After the Last Bite. Goldie Invites You on a Culinary Journey That Celebrates the Joy of Cooking and the Magic of Gathering Around the Table. Whether You're a Seasoned Chef or a Kitchen Novice, This Cookbook Promises to Be Your Trusty Companion, Sparking Creativity and Bringing a Sprinkle of Gold to Your Everyday Meals. So, Tie on Your Apron, Grab Your Favorite Wooden Spoon, and Let's Make Some Memories Together—one Delicious Dish at a Time!

Here, You'll Discover an Array of Delightful Recipes, Each Crafted With Care and a Dash of Whimsy. From Comforting Classics That Remind You of Home to Exotic Flavors That Transport You to Faraway Lands, "Goldie's Gourmet Adventures" Has Something for Everyone. Embrace the Art of Cooking With Easy-to-follow Guides Peppered With Tips and Tricks to Elevate Your Culinary Skills. As You Turn Each Page, You'll Find Stories That Capture the Essence of Food's Ability to Bring People Together— Stories of Family Gatherings, Festive Celebrations, and Quiet Moments of Joy. Join Goldie in Exploring the World of Flavors, Where Every Dish is an Adventure and Every Meal is a Celebration of Life's Simple Pleasures. With a Focus on Fresh Ingredients and Heartwarming Techniques, You're Sure to Create Dishes That Not Only Satisfy the Taste Buds but Also Warm the Soul. So, Let's Embark on This Gourmet Journey, and Make Every Meal a Memorable Experience Filled With Love and Laughter!

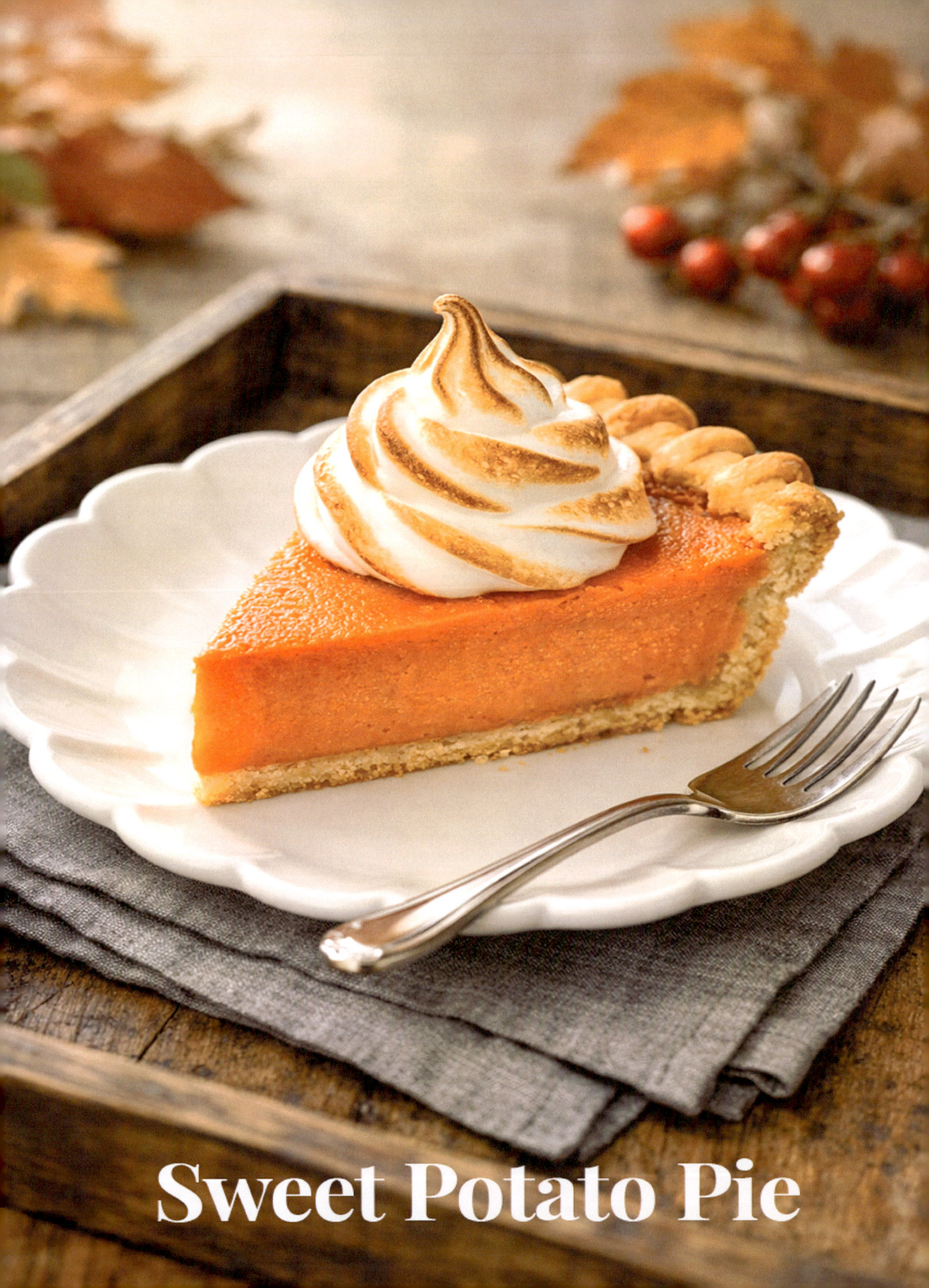
Sweet Potato Pie

Sweet Potato Pie

INSTRUCTIONS

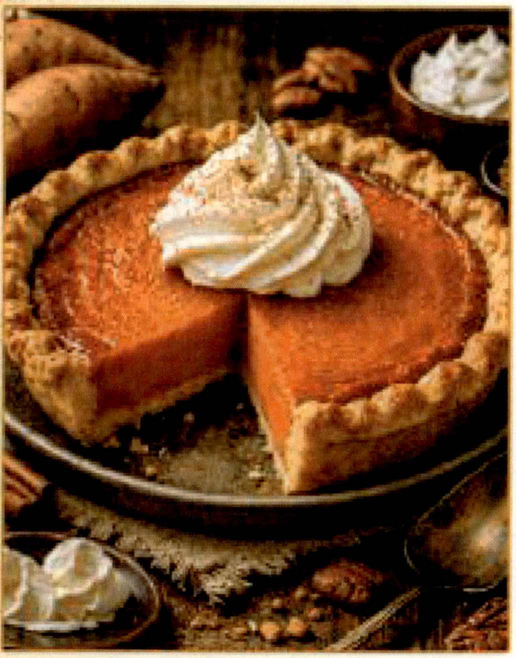

1. PREPARE THE SWEET POTATOES:
Start by Thoroughly Washing the Sweet Potatoes Under Running Water to Remove Any Dirt. Peel Them and Cut Into Chunks.

2. BOIL THE SWEET POTATOES:
Place the Sweet Potato Chunks Into a Pot of Boiling Water. Boil for About 15–20 Minutes, or Until They Are Tender and Easily Pierced With a Fork.

3. DRAIN AND COOL:
After Cooking, Drain the Sweet Potatoes and Allow Them to Cool for Approximately 15 Minutes

4. PREHEAT THE OVEN:
While the Sweet Potatoes Are Cooling, Preheat Your Oven to 350°F (175°C). Until Well Combined and Smooth.

5. MAKE THE FILLING:
In a Large Mixing Bowl, Mash the Cooled Sweet Potatoes Until Smooth. Stir in Sugar, Brown Sugar, Eggs, Milk, Vanilla Extract, Cinnamon, and Nutmeg. Mix Everything Until Well Combined and Smooth.

6. PREPARE THE PIE CRUST:
If Using a Store-bought Pie Crust, Place It in a Pie Dish. If Making Your Own, Roll Out the Dough and Fit It Into the Pie Dish, Crimping the Edges as Desired.

7. FILL THE PIE CRUST:
Pour the Sweet Potato Filling Into the Prepared Pie Crust, Spreading It Out Evenly.

8. BAKE:
Bake the Pie in the Preheated Oven for About 45–50 Minutes, or Until the Filling is Set and a Knife Inserted Into the Center Comes Out Clean.

9. COOL AND SERVE:
Once Baked, Remove the Pie From the Oven and Let It Cool on a Wire Rack. Serve Warm or at Room Temperature, and Enjoy Your Delight!

CONSIDER ADDING WHIPPED CREAM OR A SCOOP OF ICE CREAM ON TOP FOR AN EXTRA SPECIAL TREAT!

PREPARE TIME	COOK TIME
60 MINUTES	15 MINUTES

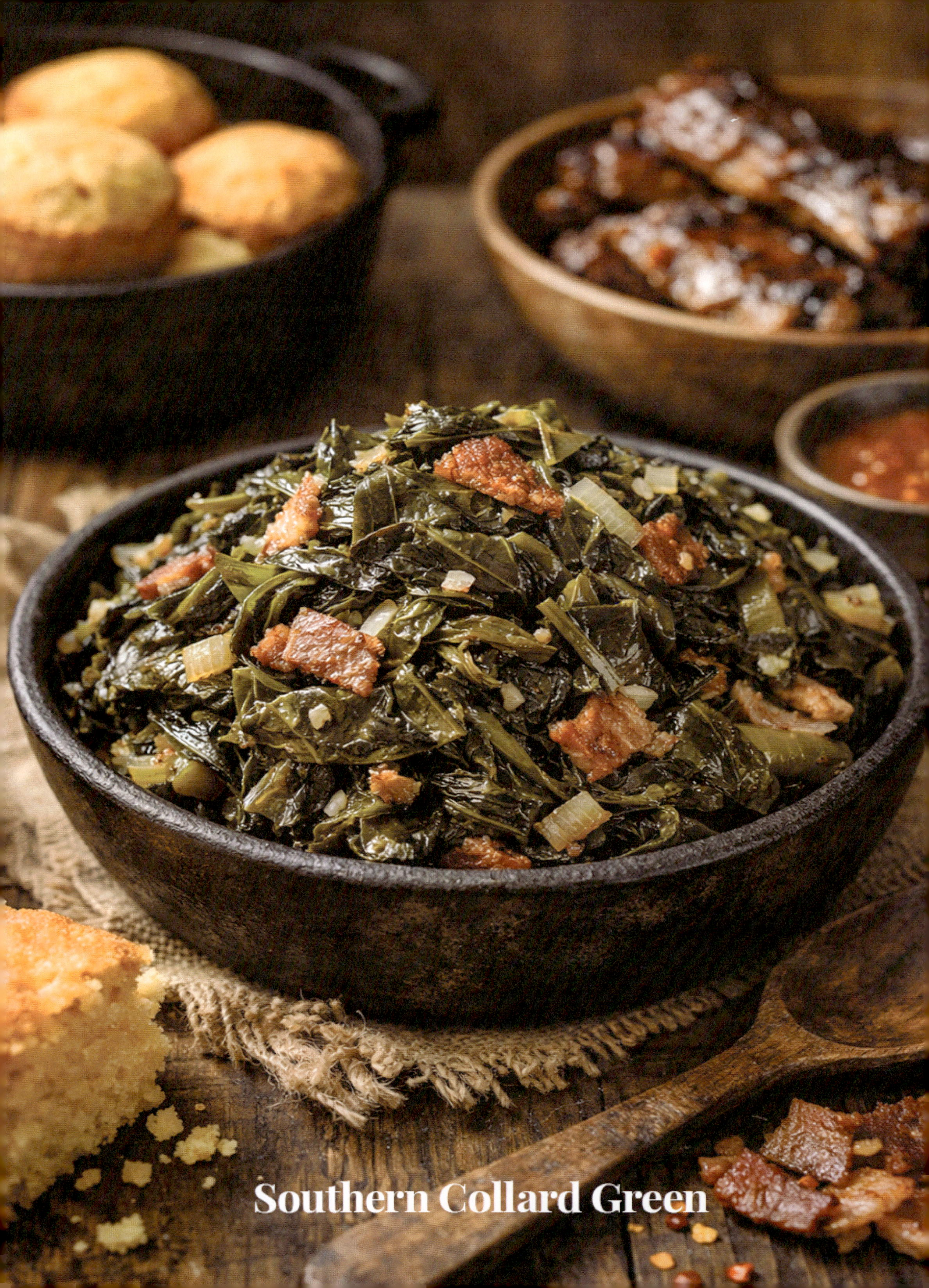

Southern Collard Green

Southern Style Collard Greens

INSTRUCTIONS

INGREDIENTS

Here Are the Ingredients You Will Need for Collard Greens:

- Collard Greens
- Olive Oil
- Salt
- Sugar (Optional, for Balancing Bitterness)
- Onion (Chopped)
- Garlic (Optional, for Added Flavor)
- Chicken or Vegetable Broth (Optional, for Cooking)
- Red Pepper Flakes (Optional, for Heat)
- Lemon Juice or Vinegar (for Serving, Optional)
- Feel Free to Adjust the Ingredients According to Your Taste!

TO PREPARE COLLARD GREENS, FOLLOW THESE

1. **WASH THE GREENS:** Start by Thoroughly Washing the Collard Greens Under Running Water to Remove Any Dirt or Grit. This is Crucial for Ensuring That They Are Clean and Safe to Eat.

2. **BOIL THE GREENS:** In a Large Pot, Bring Water to a Boil. Once Boiling, Add the Washed Collard Greens. Boil Them for About 5–10 Minutes Until They Are Tender. This Step Helps to Soften the Greens and Reduce Bitterness.

3. **SAUTÉ THE GREENS:** After Boiling, Drain the Greens and Set Them Aside. In a Large Skillet or Pan, Heat Some Oil Over Medium Heat. You Can Add Ingredients Like Garlic, Onion, or Spices to Enhance the Flavor. Sauté These Ingredients Until Fragrant.

4. **ADD THE COLLARD GREENS:** Once the Aromatics Are Ready, Add the Boiled Collard Greens to the Pan. Stir Them Into the Mixture and Sauté for Another 5–10 Minutes, Allowing the Flavors to Meld Together.

5. **SEASONING:** Add Salt, Pepper, and Any Other Seasonings You Prefer—such as Vinegar or Hot Sauce—for Added Flavor. Taste and Adjust the Seasonings as Necessary.

6. **SERVE:** Once the Collard Greens Are Well-cooked and Seasoned to Your Liking, Remove Them From Heat and Serve Them Hot as a Delicious Side Dish. Enjoy Your Collard Greens!

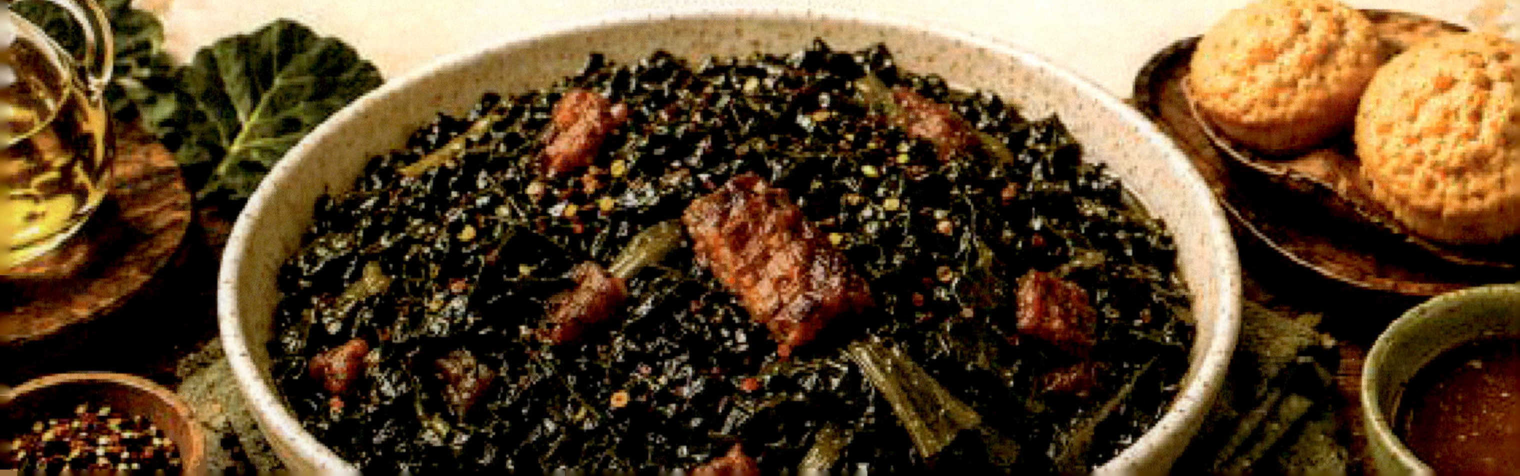

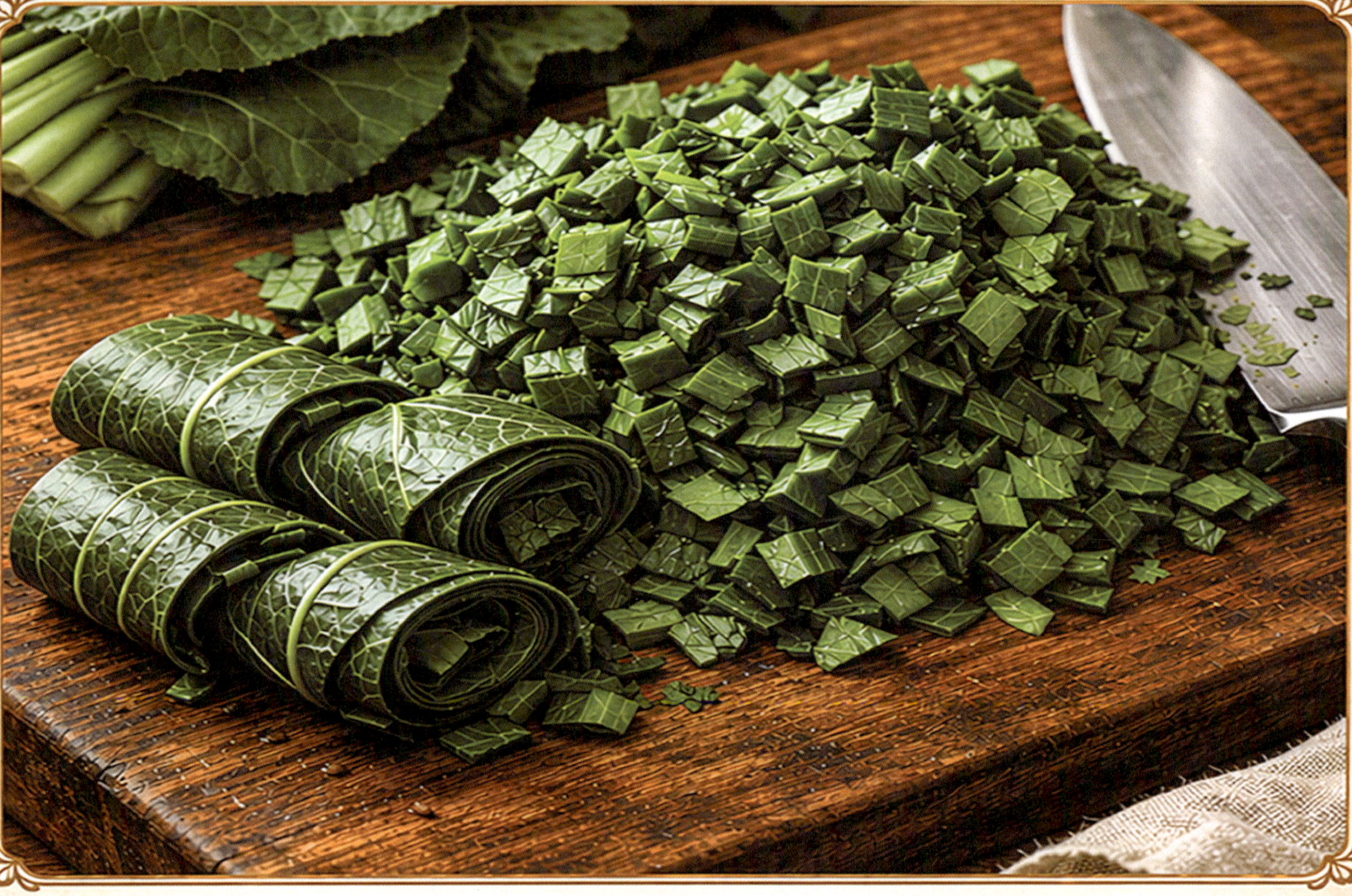

Collard Greens, a Staple in Southern Cuisine, Have a Rich History That Traces Back to Prehistoric Times. Originating From the Wild Cabbage Species Native to the Mediterranean Region, Collard Greens Have Been Cultivated for Thousands of Years. They Were Embraced by the Ancient Greeks and Romans, WHO Valued Them For Their Hardy Nature and Nutritional Benefits. Collard Greens Made Their Way to the Americas With European Settlers and Became Deeply Ingrained in Southern Food Culture, Particularly Within African American Communities. Enslaved Africans, Brought to North America, Adapted Their Culinary Traditions to Include Collard Greens, Transforming Them Into a Symbol of Resilience and Cultural Heritage. Today, Collard Greens Are Celebrated Not Only for Their Historical Significance but Also for Their Health Benefits, Being Rich in Vitamins a, C, and K, and Serving as a Beloved Dish in Both Traditional and Modern Cuisine.

Goldie Mack N Cheese

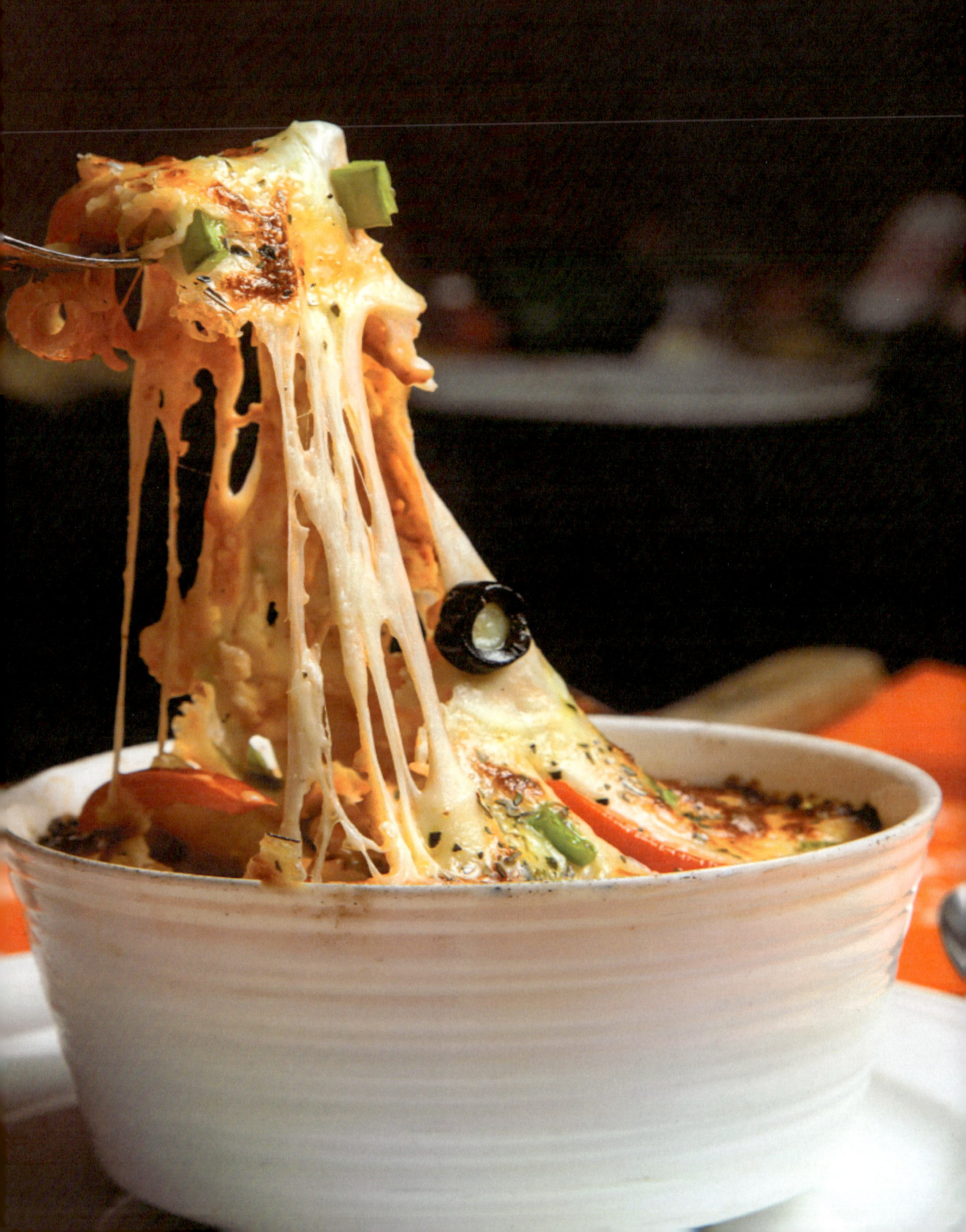

GOLDIE MACK N CHEESE

Here's a Simple and Delicious Mac and Cheese Recipe for You!

INGREDIENTS

Here Are the Ingredients You Can Use to Make a Flavorful Mac and Cheese With a Twist:

- 2 Cups Macaroni or Pasta of Your Choice
- 1 Tablespoon Olive Oil
- 1 Cup Diced Onion (You Can Use Red Onion for a Sweeter Flavor) Salt, to Taste
- 1 Teaspoon Sugar (to Balance the Flavors) 1 Cup Cooked Salmon, Flaked
- 1 Cup Shredded Cheese (Cheddar, Mozzarella, or Your Favorite Cheese
- 1 Cup Milk or Cream
- Onion Rings (for Topping)
- Feel Free to Adjust the Quantities Based on Your Preference! Enjoy Your Mac and Cheese!

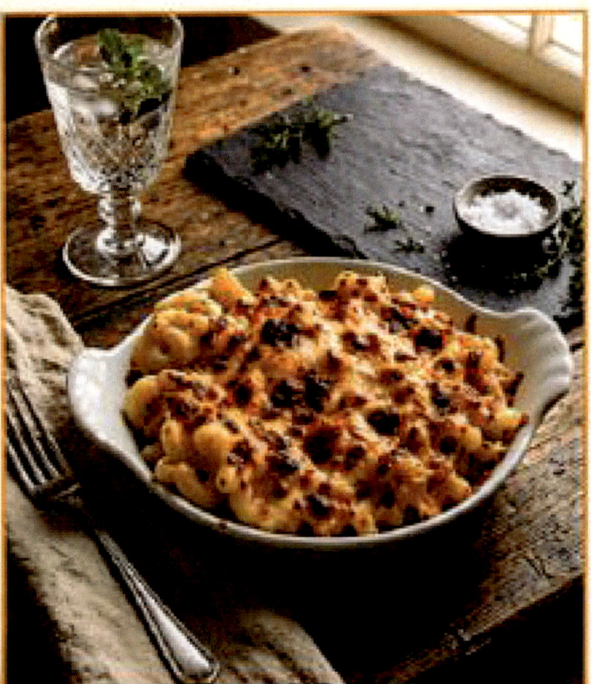

INSTRUCTIONS

1. GATHER THE FOLLOWING INGREDIENTS:

- 8 Ounces of Elbow Macaroni
- 2 Cups of Shredded Sharp Cheddar Cheese 1/2 Cup of Grated Parmesan Cheese 3 Cups of Milk
- 1/4 Cup of Butter
- 2 1/2 Tablespoons of All-purpose Flour Salt and Pepper to Taste
- Optional: Breadcrumbs for Topping

2. COOK THE PASTA:

- In a Large Pot, Bring Salted Water to a Boil.
- Add the Elbow Macaroni and Cook According to the Package Instructions Until Al Dente. Drain and Set Aside.

3. MAKE THE CHEESE SAUCE:

- In the Same Pot, Melt the Butter Over Medium Heat.
- Stir in the Flour to Create a Roux, Cooking for About 1-2 Minutes Until It's Lightly Golden
- Gradually Whisk in the Milk, Ensuring There Are No Lumps. Continue to Stir Until the Mixture Thickens, About 5-7 Minutes.
- Add the Shredded Cheddar and Grated Parmesan Cheese to the Sauce, Stirring Until Melted and Smooth. Season With Salt and Pepper.

4. COMBINE:

- Add the Cooked Macaroni to the Cheese Sauce, Stirring Until Well Combined.

5. OPTIONAL BAKING STEP:

- If You Like a Crispy Topping, Preheat Your Oven to 350°F (175°C).
- Transfer the Mac and Cheese to a Baking Dish, Sprinkle With Breadcrumbs, and Bake for About 20 Minutes Until Golden and Bubbly.

6. SERVE:

- Let It Cool for a Few Minutes Before Serving. Enjoy Your Homemade Mac and Cheese!

Feel Free to Customize With Spices or Add-ins Like Cooked Bacon, Vegetables, or Different Types of Cheese!

Honey BBQ Wings

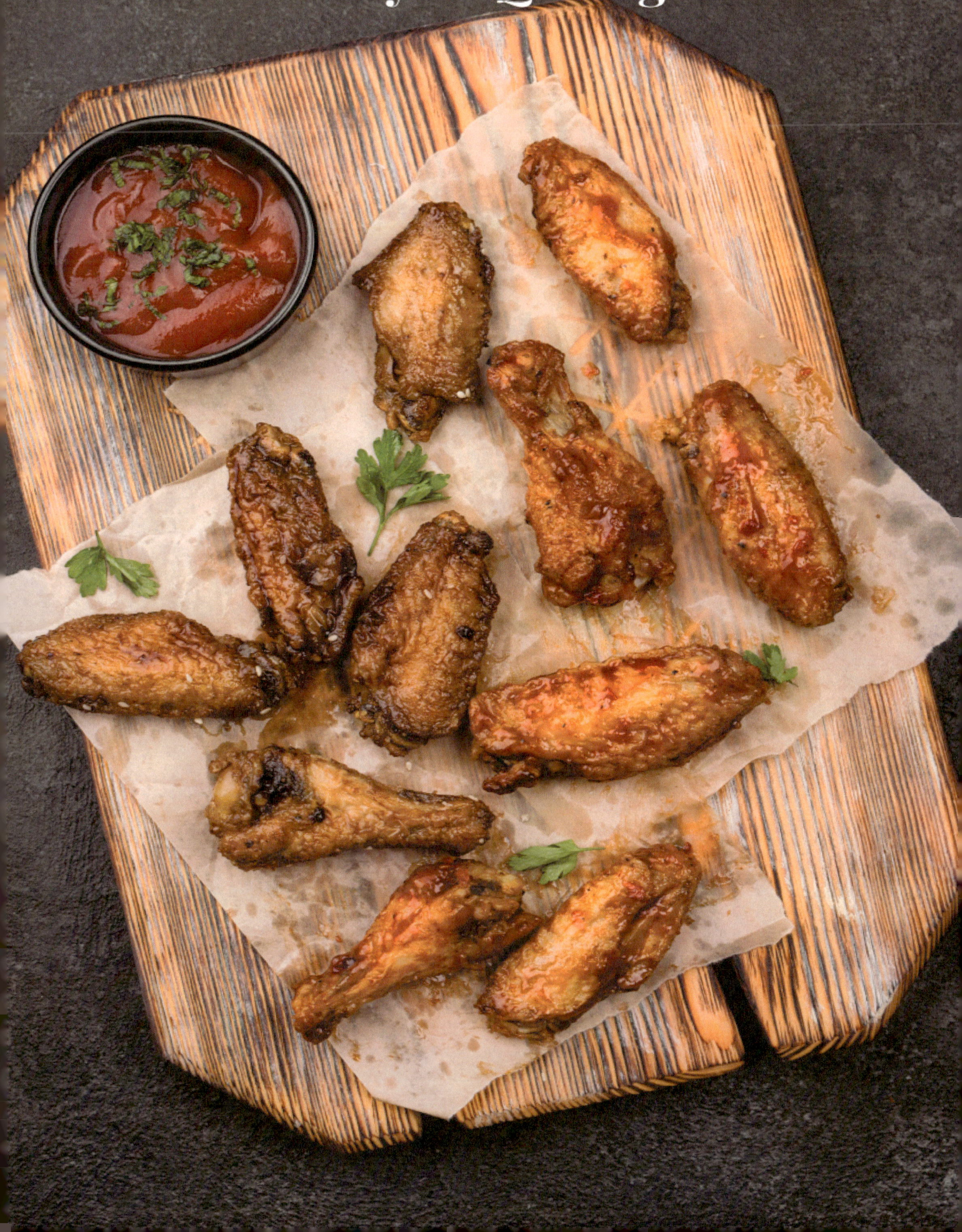

HONEY BBQ WINGS

Here's a Step-by-step Guide to Making Delicious Fried Honey Bbq Wings:

INGREDIENTS

- Chicken Wings: 2
- Honey: 1/4 Cup
- Bbq Sauce: 1/2 Cup
- Salt: 1 Teaspoon (or to taste)
- Pepper: 1/2 Teaspoon (or to taste)
- Garlic Powder: 1 Teaspoon
- Onion Powder: 1 Teaspoon
- Oil For Frying: Enough to Submerge The Wings (Approximately 2–3 cups, depending on the frying method)
- Feel Free To Adjust The Quantities Based On Your Taste Preferences!

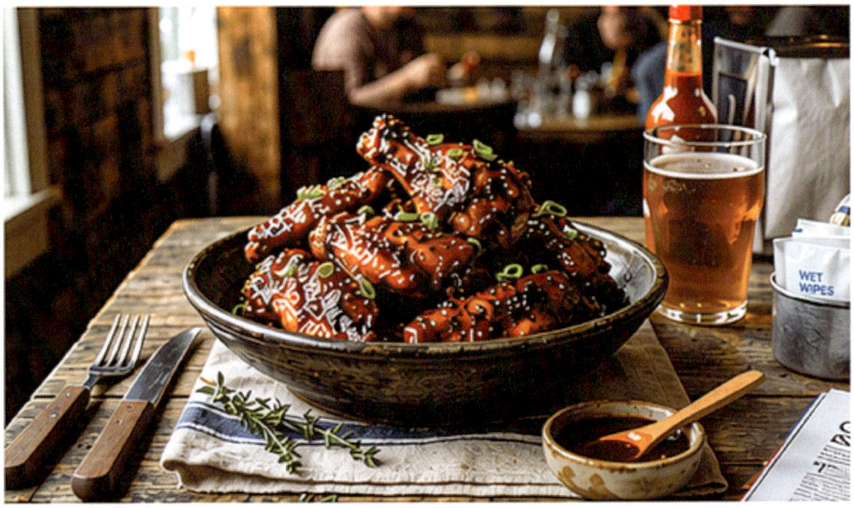

PREPARE TIME: **15 MINUTES** | COOK TIME: **40 MINUTES** | SERVE TIME: **5 MINUTES**

INSTRUCTIONS

1. PREPARE THE WINGS:

- Start by Thoroughly Washing the Chicken Wings Under Cold Running Water. This Helps Remove Any Surface

2. DRY THE WINGS:

- Pat the Wings Dry With Paper Towels. This Step is Important for Achieving a Crispy Texture When Frying.

3. MARINATE:

- In a Large Bowl, Mix Honey, Bbq Sauce, Salt, Pepper, Garlic Powder, and Onion Powder to Create a Marinade.
- Add the Chicken Wings to the Marinade, Ensuring They Are Well-Coated. Let Them Marinate for at Least 30 Minutes for Better Flavor (You Can Refrigerate Them for a Few Hours or Overnight for Even More Flavor).

4. HEAT THE OIL:

- In a Large Pot or Deep Fryer, Heat Oil to Around 350°F (175°C). You'll Need Enough Oil to Fully Submerge the Wings.

5. FRY THE WINGS:

- Carefully Add the Marinated Wings to the Hot Oil in Batches, Being Careful Not to Overcrowd the Pot. Fry for About 8–10 Minutes or Until Golden Brown and Cooked Through (Internal Temperature Should Reach 165°F / 74°C).
- Use a Slotted Spoon to Remove the Wings and Place Them on a Paper Towel-lined Plate to Drain Excess Oil.

6. COAT WITH SAUCE:

- In a Clean Bowl, Mix Some Additional Bbq Sauce With Honey. Toss the Fried Wings in This Sauce Mixture Until They Are Well-coated.

7. SERVE:

- Serve the Wings Hot, Garnished With Chopped Green Onions or Sesame Seeds if Desired. Enjoy Your Fried Honey Bbq Wings With Your Favorite Dipping Sauces!

Remember to Maintain Cleanliness Throughout the Cooking Process and Enjoy Your Delicious Wings!

Not Grandmas Banana Pudding

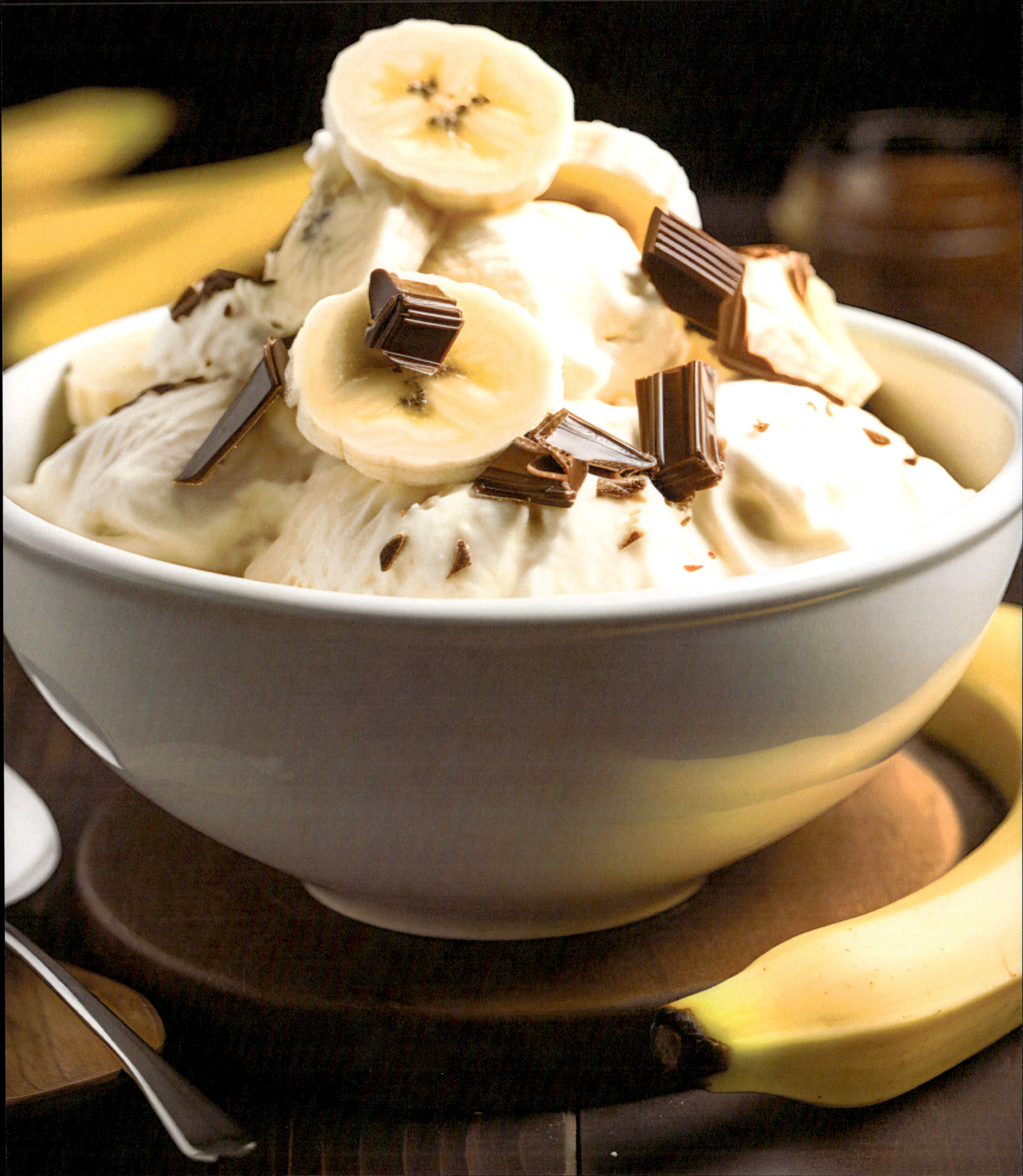

Not Grandmas Banana Pudding

Cook Time:
4 to 6 Hours

Prepare Time:
15 Minutes

Serve Time:
30 minutes

Instructions

To Make Banana Pudding:

1. **Gather Ingredients:** Ripe Bananas, Vanilla Pudding Mix, Milk, Vanilla Wafers, Whipped Cream.
2. **Prepare Pudding:** Mix Pudding Mix With Milk, Whisk Until Smooth, and Let Thicken.
3. **Slice Bananas:** Peel and Cut Bananas Into Thin Rounds.
4. **Layer Ingredients:** In a Dish, Layer Vanilla Wafers, Bananas, and Pudding Repeatedly, Ending With Pudding.
5. **Top It Off:** Add Whipped Cream and Optionally Crushed Vanilla Wafers.
6. **Chill:** Cover and Refrigerate for at Least 2 Hours.

Ingredients

To prepare a classic banana pudding, you will typically need the following ingredients along with their measurements:

- 4 cups of milk
- 3/4 cup of granulated sugar
- 1/4 cup of brown sugar
- 1/4 teaspoon of salt
- 1/2 cup of all-purpose flour
- 1 teaspoon of vanilla extract
- 4 ripe bananas, sliced
- 1 box (about 11 ounces) of vanilla wafers
- 2 cups of whipped cream or meringue for topping

Feel Free to Adjust the Quantities Based on Your Taste Preferences or Serving Size. Enjoy Your Cooking!

Serve: Enjoy Chilled Banana Pudding!

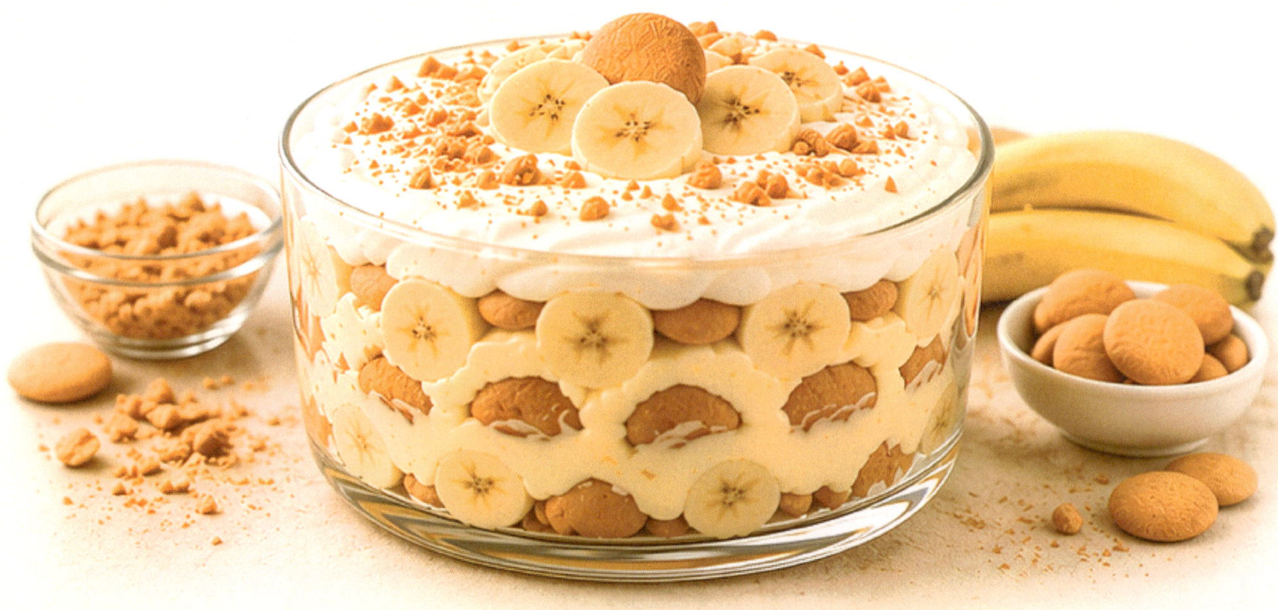

Strawberry Crunch Cheesecake

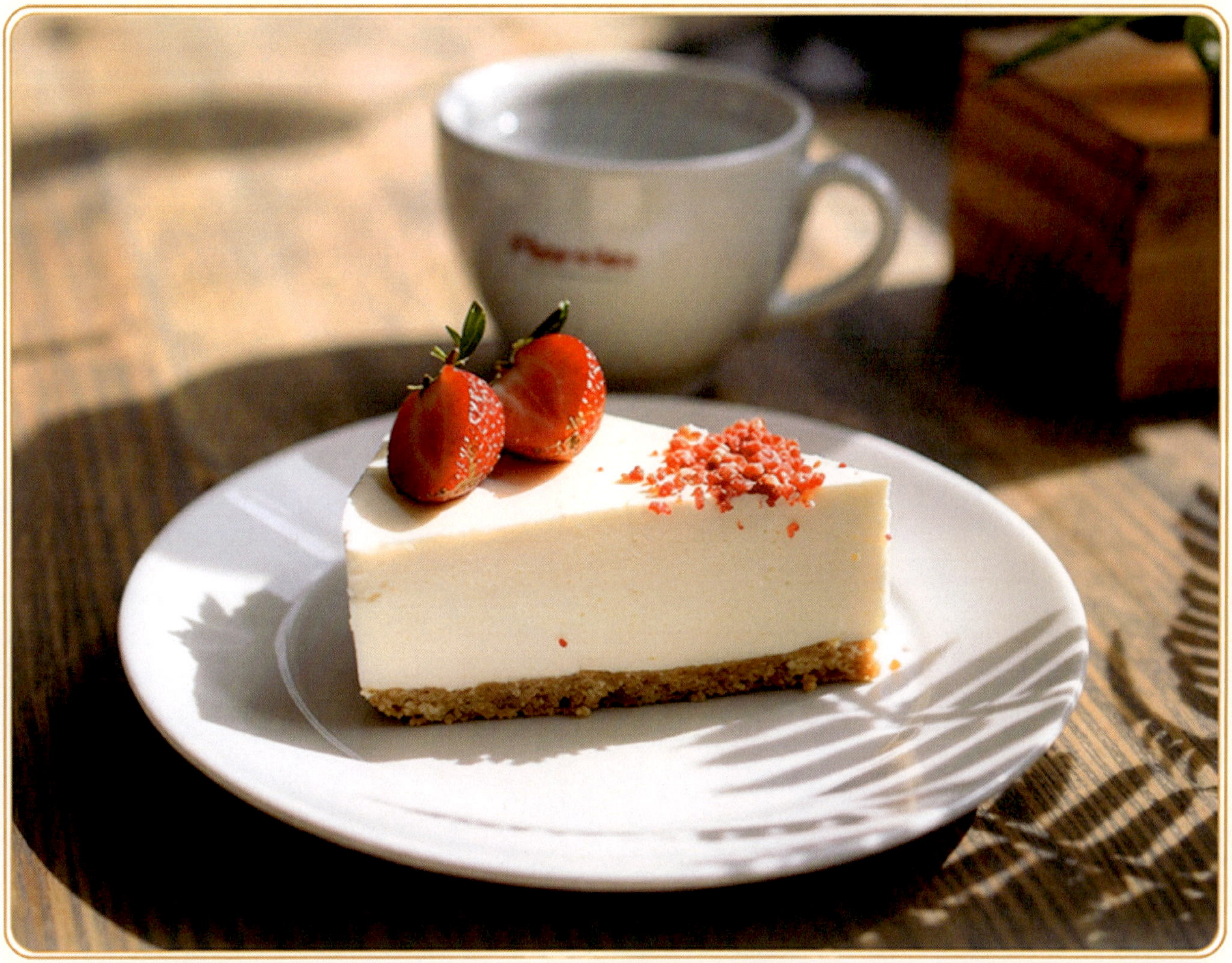

Strawberry cheesecake has a rich history, originating in ancient Greece where cheesecake made with fresh cheese and honey was served to athletes. It evolved over time, particularly in the U.S. with the introduction of cream cheese in the 1870s. The addition of strawberries enhanced its flavor and visual appeal, leading to its popularity as a favorite dessert. Today, it is cherished for its creamy texture and sweet-tart balance, often featured at gatherings and special occasions, representing a blend of tradition and innovation in desserts.

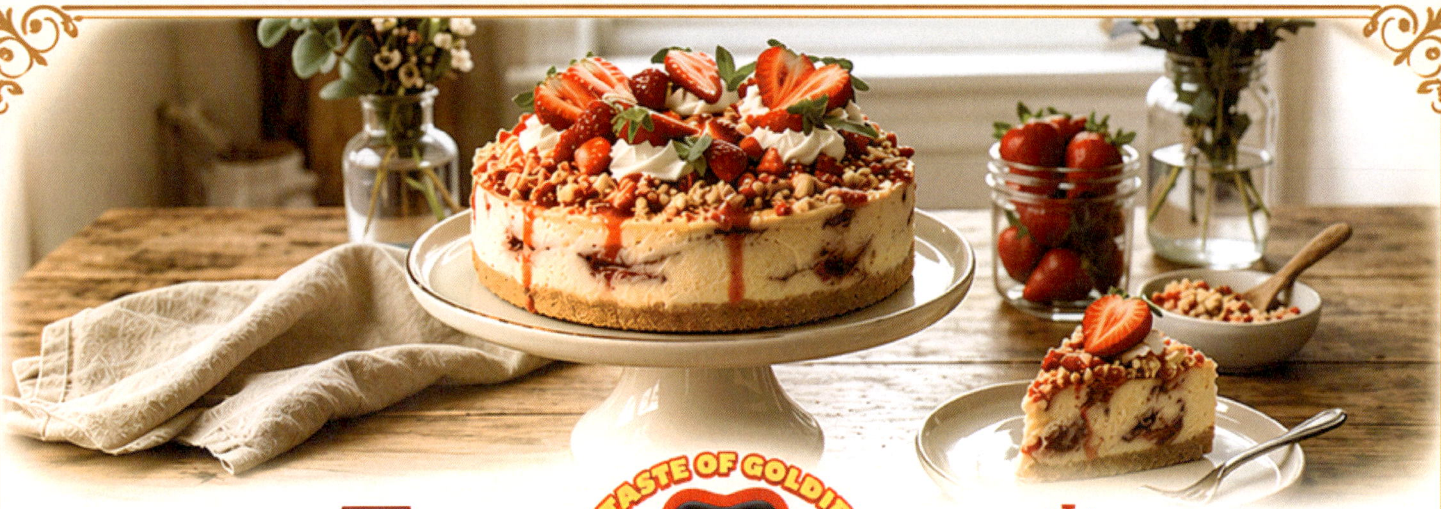

PREPARE TIME
15 MINUTES

COOK TIME
1 HOUR

STRAWBERRY CRUNCH CHEESECAKE

INSTRUCTIONS

1. INGREDIENT PREPARATION:

- Gather the Necessary Ingredients: Cream Cheese, Sugar, Vanilla Extract, Sour Cream, Eggs, and Fresh Strawberries.
- Wash the Strawberries Thoroughly and Remove Their Stems.

2. CRUST PREPARATION:

- Mix Crushed Graham Crackers With Melted Butter and a Sprinkle of Sugar in a Bowl.
- Firmly Press This Mixture Into the Bottom of a Springform Pan to Create the Crust.

3. CHEISECAKE FILLING:

- Beat the Cream Cheese in a Mixing Bowl Until Creamy.
- Gradually Add Sugar and Vanilla Extract, Mixing Until Well Blended.
- Fold in the Sour Cream and Continue to Beat Until Smooth.
- Add the Eggs ONE at a Time, Mixing Gently After Each Addition Until Just Blended.

4. COMBINE AND BAKE:

- Pour the Cheesecake Filling Over the Prepared Crust in the Springform Pan
- Bake in a Preheated Oven at 325°F (160°C) for Approximately 50–60 Minutes, or Until the Center is Set but Still Slightly Wobbly.

INGREDIENTS

To Make a Delicious Strawberry Cheesecake, Follow These Steps:

- Crust:
- 1½ Cups Graham Cracker Crumbs
- ½ Cup Unsalted Butter (Melted)
- ¼ Cup Granulated Sugar
- Filling:
- 4 (8-ounce) Packages Cream Cheese (Softened)
- 1 Cup Granulated Sugar
- 1 Teaspoon Vanilla Extract
- 4 Large Eggs
- 1 Cup Sour Cream
- 1 Cup Heavy Cream
- STRAWBERRY TOPPING:
- 2 Cups Fresh Strawberries (Hulled and Sliced)
- ¼ Cup Granulated Sugar
- 1 Tablespoon Lemon Juice

5. STRAWBERRY TOPPING:

- While the Cheesecake is Baking, Slice the Cleaned Strawberries and Mix Them With a Bit of Sugar to Enhance Their Flavor.
- Allow Them to Sit for About 10–15 Minutes to Release Their Juices.

6. CHILL AND SERVE:

- Once the Cheesecake Has Finished Baking, Let It Cool to Room Temperature Before Refrigerating for at Least 4 Hours or Overnight.
- After Chilling, Top the Cheesecake With the Macerated Strawberries Just Before Serving.

ENJOY YOUR HOMEMADE STRAWBERRY CHEESECAKE!

Rotel Dip

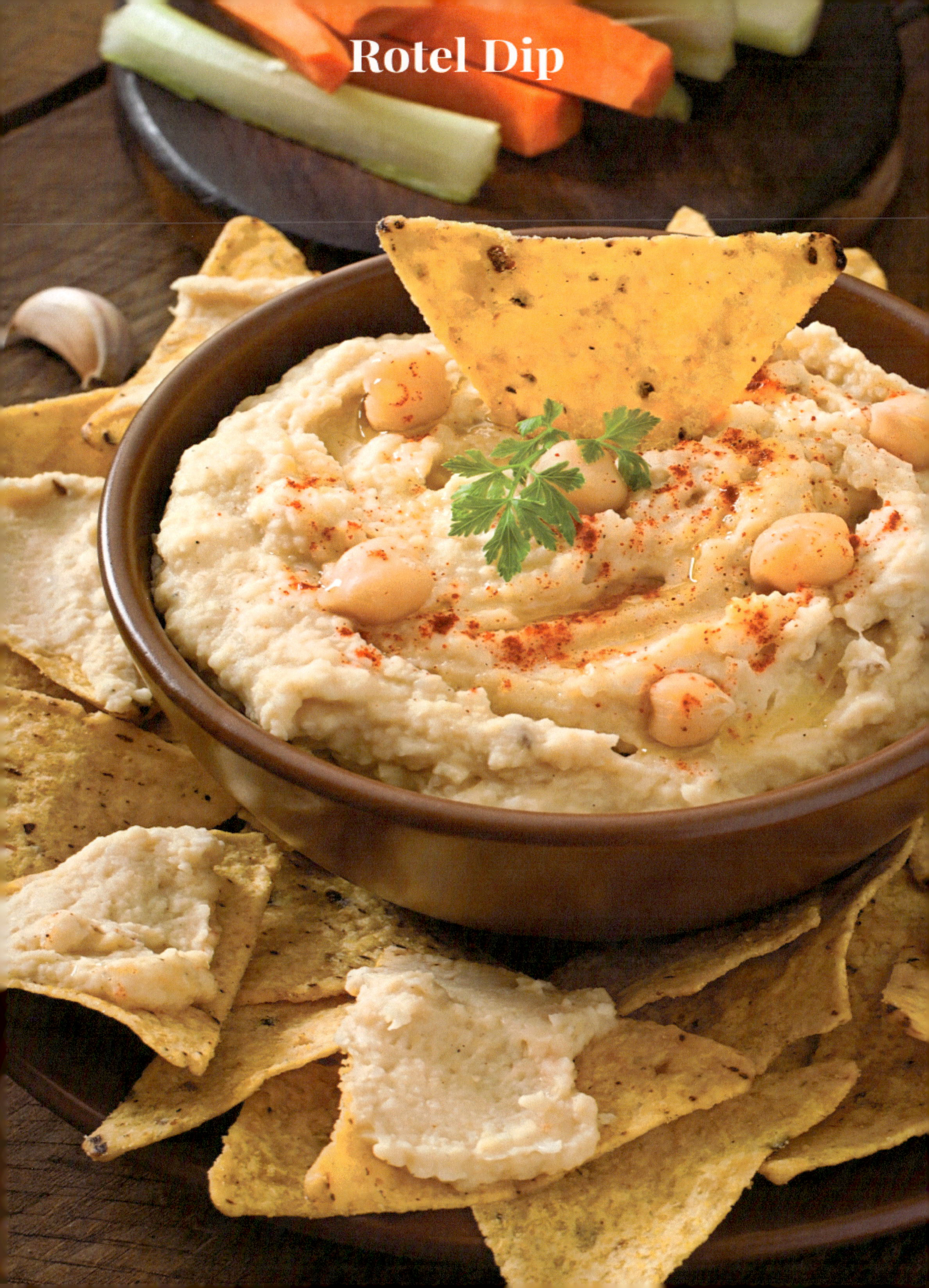

Rotel Dip

Instructions

1. **Brown the Meat:** In a skillet over medium heat, cook the ground beef or sausage until fully browned. Drain any excess fat.

2. **Combine Ingredients:** Lower the heat to medium-low. Add the cubed Velveeta cheese and can of Rotel tomatoes (do not drain) to the skillet with the meat. Stir occasionally until the cheese is completely melted and the mixture is smooth.

3. **Adjust Seasoning:** Taste and add salt or pepper if needed. You can also stir in additional ingredients like chopped onions or jalapeños for extra flavor.

4. **Serve:** Transfer the dip to a serving bowl. Garnish with cilantro if desired. Serve warm with tortilla chips, crackers, or vegetables.

Ingredients

- 1 Pound Ground Beef or Sausage
- 1 Can (10 Oz) Rotel Diced Tomatoes and Green Chilies
- 1 Block (16 Oz) Velveeta Cheese, Cubed
- Optional: Chopped Onions, Jalapeños, or Cilantro for Garnish

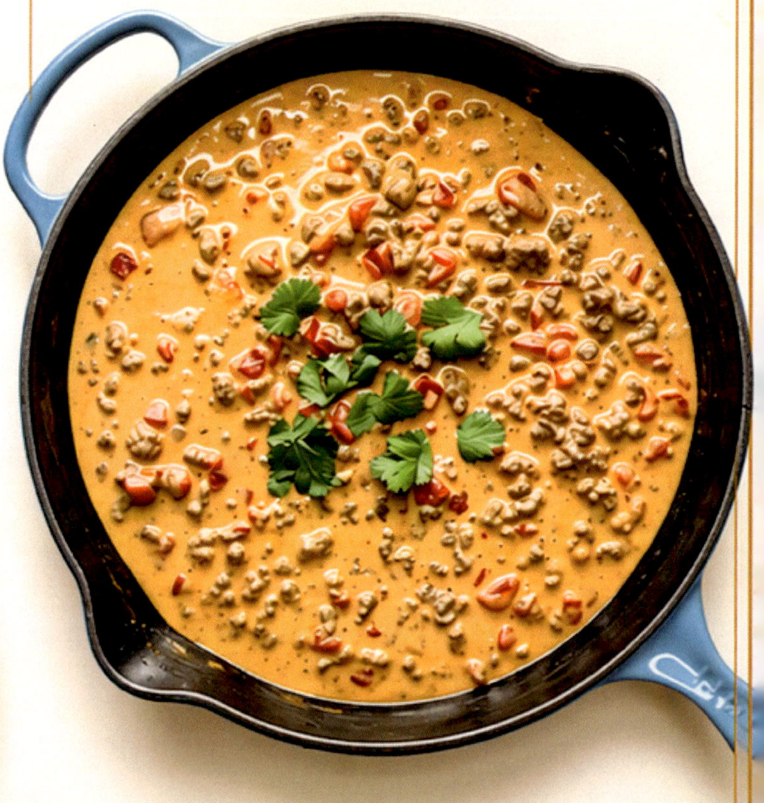

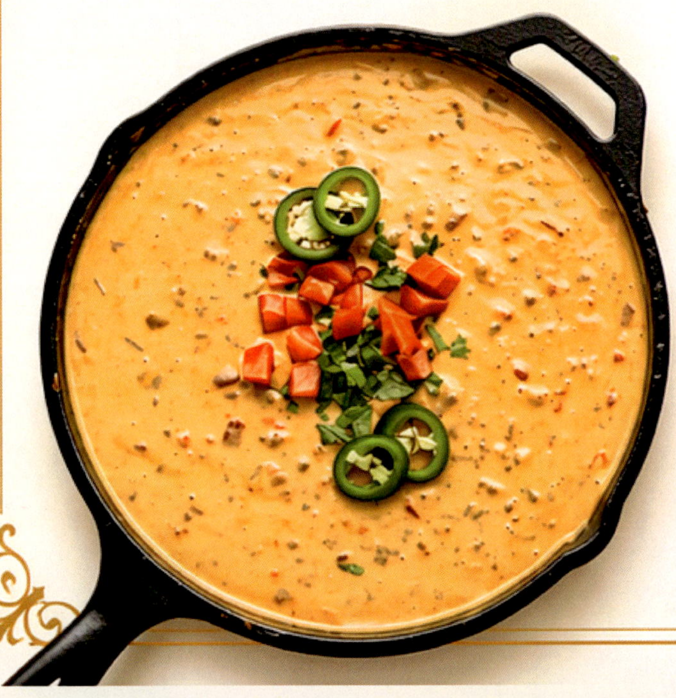

Philly Cheese Steak Eggrolls

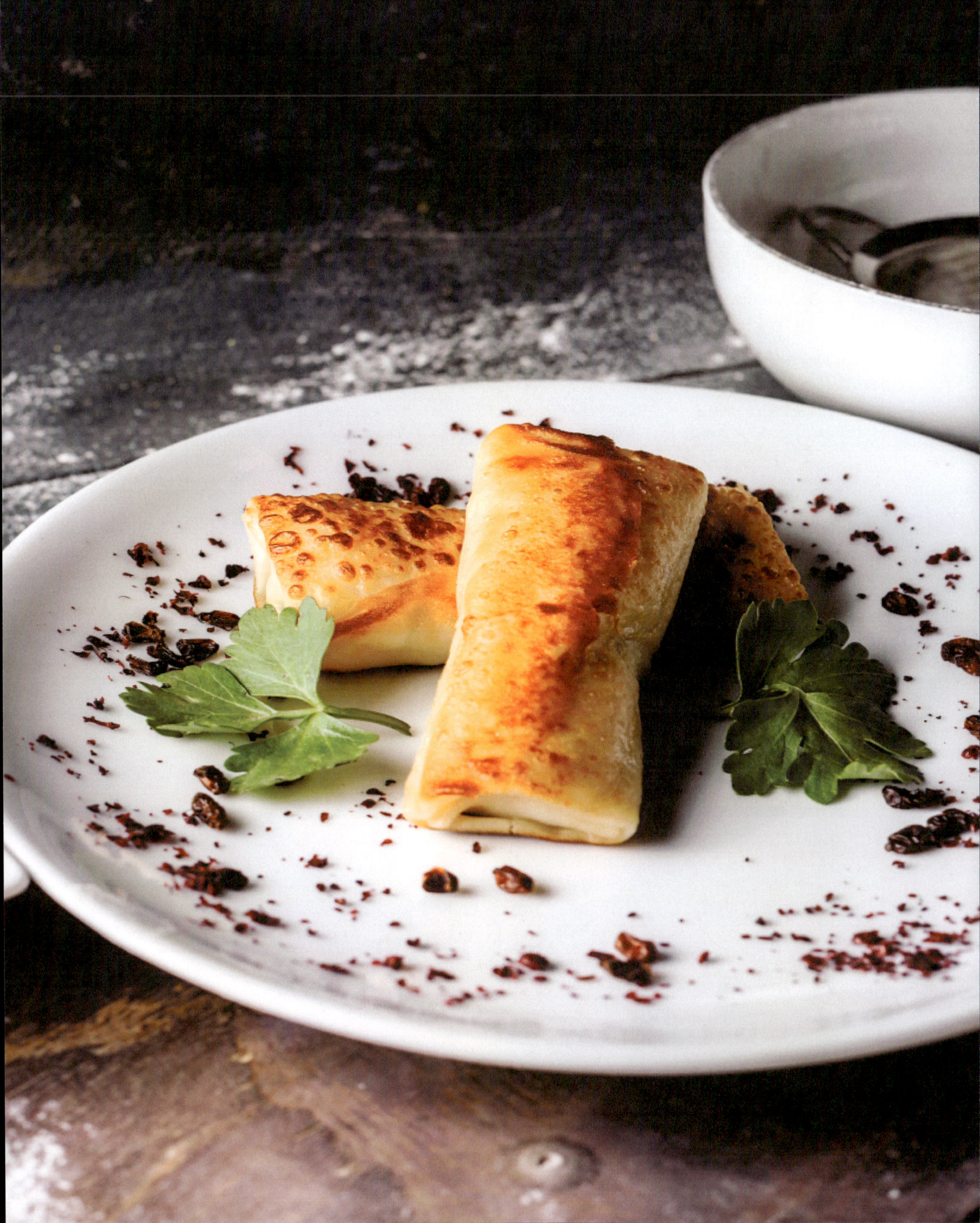

PHILLY CHEESE STEAK EGGROLLS

INSTRUCTIONS

1. PREPARE THE FILLING:

- Heat Vegetable Oil in a Large Skillet Over Medium–High Heat. Add the Ribeye Steak and Cook Until Browned, About 3–4 Minutes. Remove From Skillet and Set Aside.
- In the Same Skillet, Add Onions, Bell Peppers, and Mushrooms (if Using). Sauté Until They Are Tender, About 5 Minutes.
- Return the Steak to the Skillet, Add Garlic Powder, Salt, and Pepper. Stir to Combine and Cook for an Additional 2 Minutes. Remove From Heat and Let Cool Slightly.

2. ASSEMBLE THE EGG ROLLS:

- Lay an Egg Roll Wrapper on a Clean Surface, With a Corner Pointing Towards You. Place a Slice of Provolone Cheese in the Center of the Wrapper.
- Spoon About 2 Tablespoons of the Steak Mixture Onto the Cheese.
- Fold the Bottom Corner of the Wrapper Over the Filling, Then Fold in the Sides. Roll Tightly Towards the Top Corner, Sealing the Edge With a Dab of Water.

INGREDIENTS

- 1 Lb Thinly Sliced Ribeye Steak
- 1 Tablespoon Vegetable Oil
- 1 Medium Onion, Thinly Sliced
- 1 Green Bell Pepper, Thinly Sliced
- 1 Cup Mushrooms, Sliced (Optional)
- 1 Teaspoon Garlic Powder
- Salt and Pepper to Taste
- 8 Slices Provolone Cheese
- 12 Egg Roll Wrappers
- Oil for Frying

3. FRY THE EGG ROLLS:

- Heat Oil in a Deep Fryer or Large Pot to 350°F (175°C).
- Carefully Place Egg Rolls in the Hot Oil, a Few at a Time, and Fry Until Golden Brown and Crispy, About 3–4 Minutes.
- Remove With a Slotted Spoon and Drain on Paper Towels.

4. SERVE:

- Serve the Egg Rolls Hot With Your Choice of Dipping Sauce, Such as a Creamy Horseradish or Spicy Mustard.

ENJOY YOUR DELICIOUS PHILLY CHEESESTEAK EGG ROLLS!

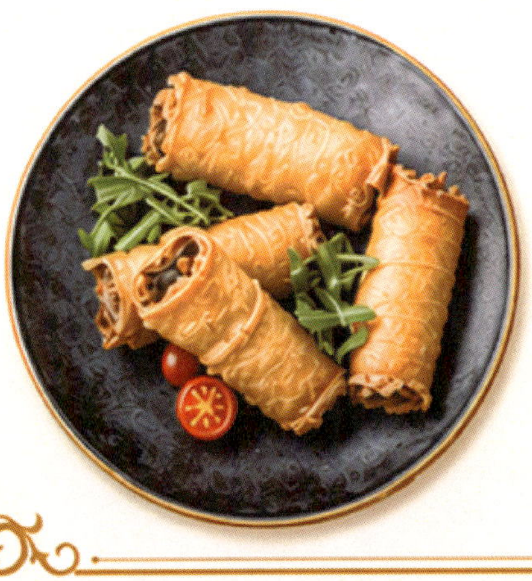

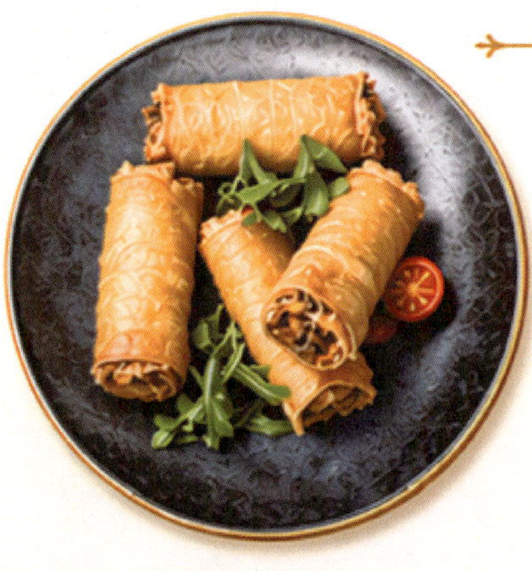

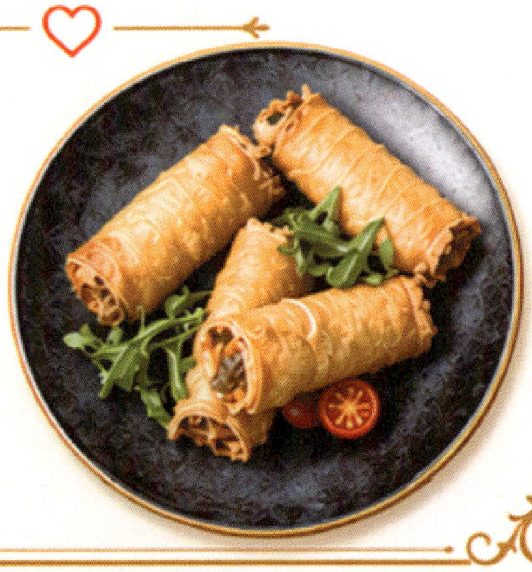

Peach Cobbler

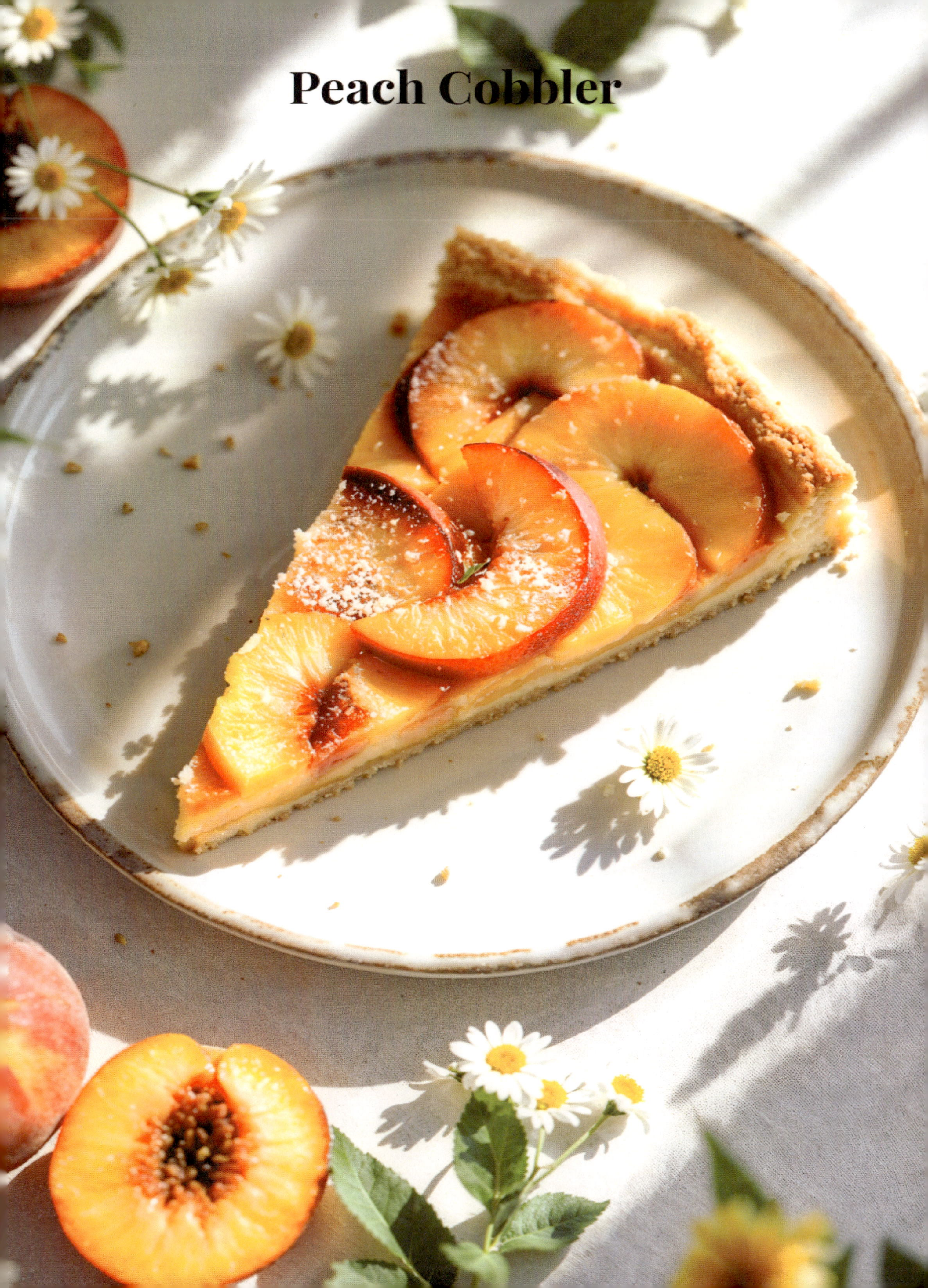

PEACH COBBLER

Here's a Delicious Recipe for Peach Cobbler:

INSTRUCTIONS

1. PREHEAT THE OVEN:

- Preheat Your Oven to 375°F (190°C).

2. PREPARE THE PEACHES:

- In a Large Bowl, Combine the Sliced Peaches, 1/2 Cup of Granulated Sugar, Brown Sugar, Salt, Cinnamon, Nutmeg, Lemon Juice, and Cornstarch. Mix Well Until the Peaches Are Evenly Coated.

3. COOK THE PEACH FILLING:

- Transfer the Peach Mixture to a Large Saucepan and Cook Over Medium Heat for About 5 Minutes, Until the Juices Thicken Slightly. Remove From Heat and Set Aside.

4. MAKE THE BATTER:

- In Another Bowl, Whisk Together the Flour, Remaining 1/2 Cup of Granulated Sugar, and Baking Powder. Stir in the Melted Butter and Milk Until You Have a Smooth Batter.

5. ASSEMBLE THE COBBLER:

- Pour the Batter Into a Greased 9x13-inch Baking Dish. Spoon the Peach Mixture Evenly Over the Batter. Do Not Stir; the Batter Will Rise Around the Peaches as It Bakes.

6. BAKE:

- Bake in the Preheated Oven for 35-40 Minutes, or Until the Top is Golden Brown and the Filling is Bubbly.

INGREDIENTS

FOR THE CAKE:

- 6 to 8 Fresh Peaches, Peeled and Sliced
- 1 Cup Granulated Sugar, Divided
- 1/2 Cup Brown Sugar
- 1/4 Teaspoon Salt
- 1 Teaspoon Ground Cinnamon
- 1/4 Teaspoon Ground Nutmeg
- 1 Tablespoon Lemon Juice
- 2 Teaspoons Cornstarch
- 1 Cup All-purpose Flour
- 1 Tablespoon Baking Powder
- 1/2 Cup Unsalted Butter, Melted
- 1 Cup Milk
- Vanilla ICE Cream or Whipped Cream for Serving (Optional)

FOR THE GLAZE:

- 1 Cup Powdered Sugar
- 2 Tablespoons Milk
- 1 Teaspoon Vanilla Extract

7. SERVE:

- Allow the Cobbler to Cool Slightly Before Serving. Enjoy It Warm With a Scoop of Vanilla ICE Cream or a Dollop of Whipped Cream, if Desired.

Enjoy Your Homemade Peach Cobbler!

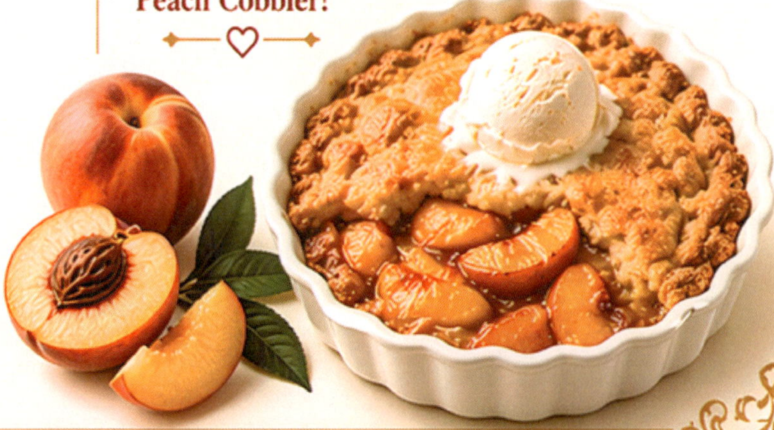

Cheer Wine Pound Cake

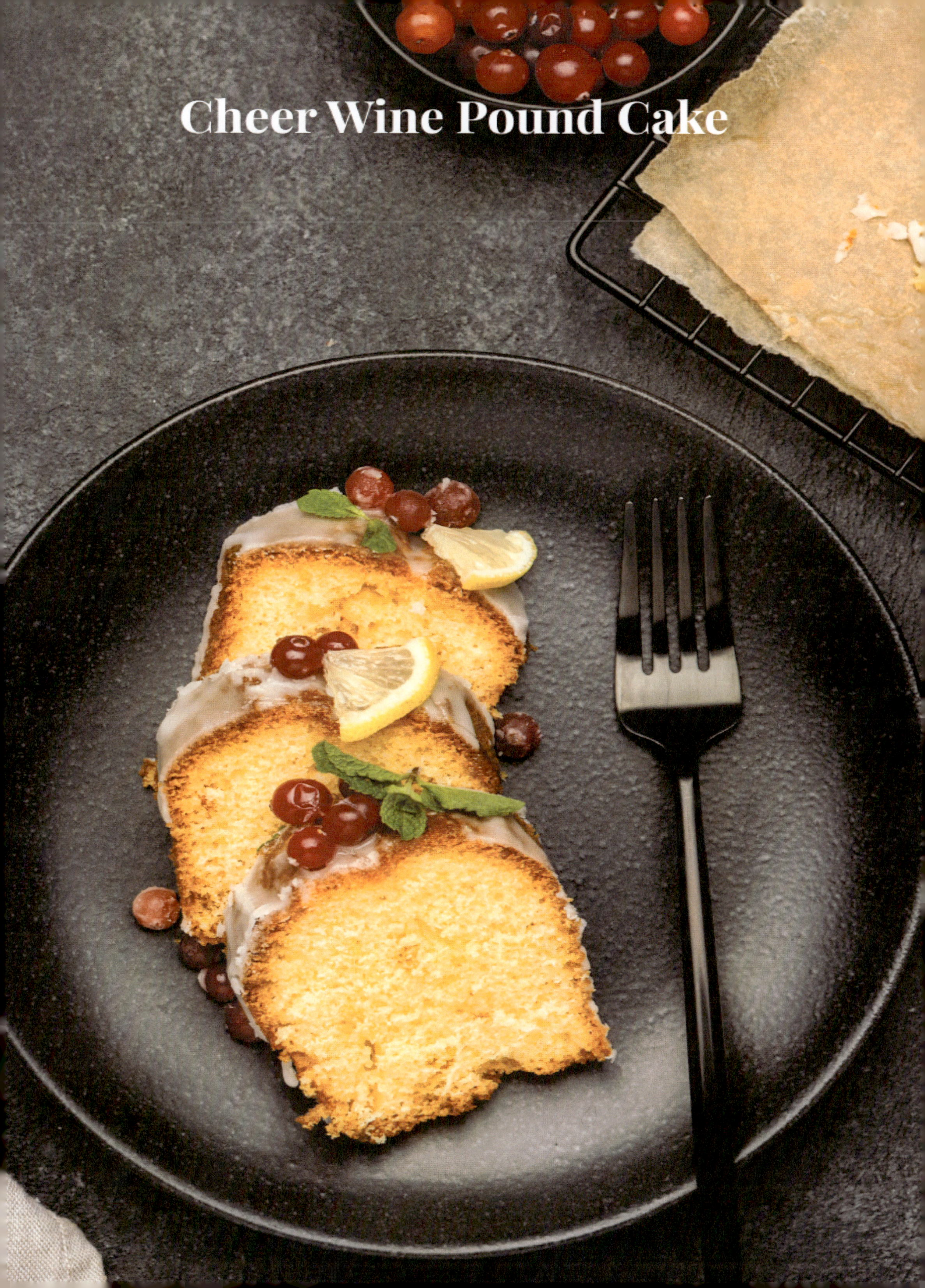

Cheer Wine Pound Cake

Here's a Delicious Recipe for Peach Cobbler:

Instructions

1. **PREHEAT THE OVEN:** Preheat your oven to 325°F (165°C). Grease and flour a 10-inch Bundt pan.

2. **MIX DRY INGREDIENTS:** In a medium bowl, whisk together the flour, baking powder, and salt. Set aside.

3. **CREAM BUTTER AND SUGAR:** In a large bowl, beat the softened butter with an electric mixer on medium speed until creamy. Gradually add the sugar, continuing to beat until light and fluffy.

4. **ADD EGGS AND VANILLA:** Add the eggs one at a time, beating well after each addition. Mix in the vanilla extract.

5. **COMBINE CHEERWINE AND BUTTERMILK:** In a separate small bowl, combine the Cheerwine soda and buttermilk. If desired, add a few drops of red food coloring for a more vibrant color.

6. **ALTERNATE ADDING FLOUR AND LIQUID:** Gradually add the flour mixture to the creamed butter mixture, alternating with the Cheerwine and buttermilk mixture. Begin and end with the flour mixture, mixing until just combined after each addition.

7. **POUR AND BAKE:** Pour the batter into the prepared Bundt pan and smooth the top with a spatula. Bake for 60–70 minutes, or until a toothpick inserted into the center comes out clean.

Ingredients

- 2 Cups All-purpose Flour
- 1/2 Teaspoon Baking Powder
- 1/4 Teaspoon Salt
- 1 Cup Unsalted Butter, Softened
- 2 Cups Granulated Sugar
- 4 Large Eggs
- 1 Teaspoon Vanilla Extract
- 1/2 Cup Cheerwine Soda
- 1/2 Cup Buttermilk
- Red Food Coloring (Optional)

8. **COOL AND SERVE:** Allow the cake to cool in the pan for about 15 minutes before inverting it onto a wire rack to cool completely. Slice and serve, enjoying the unique flavor of Cheerwine in every bite!

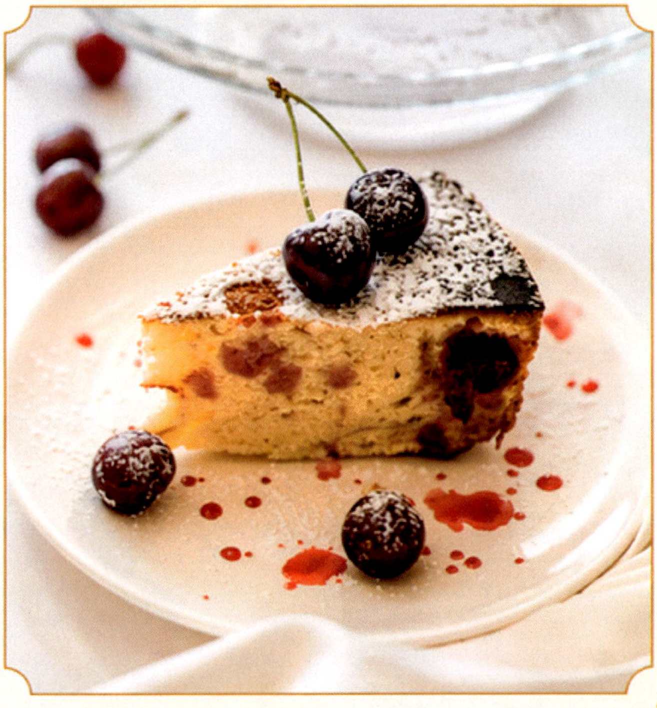

Pear Infused BBQ Lamb Chops

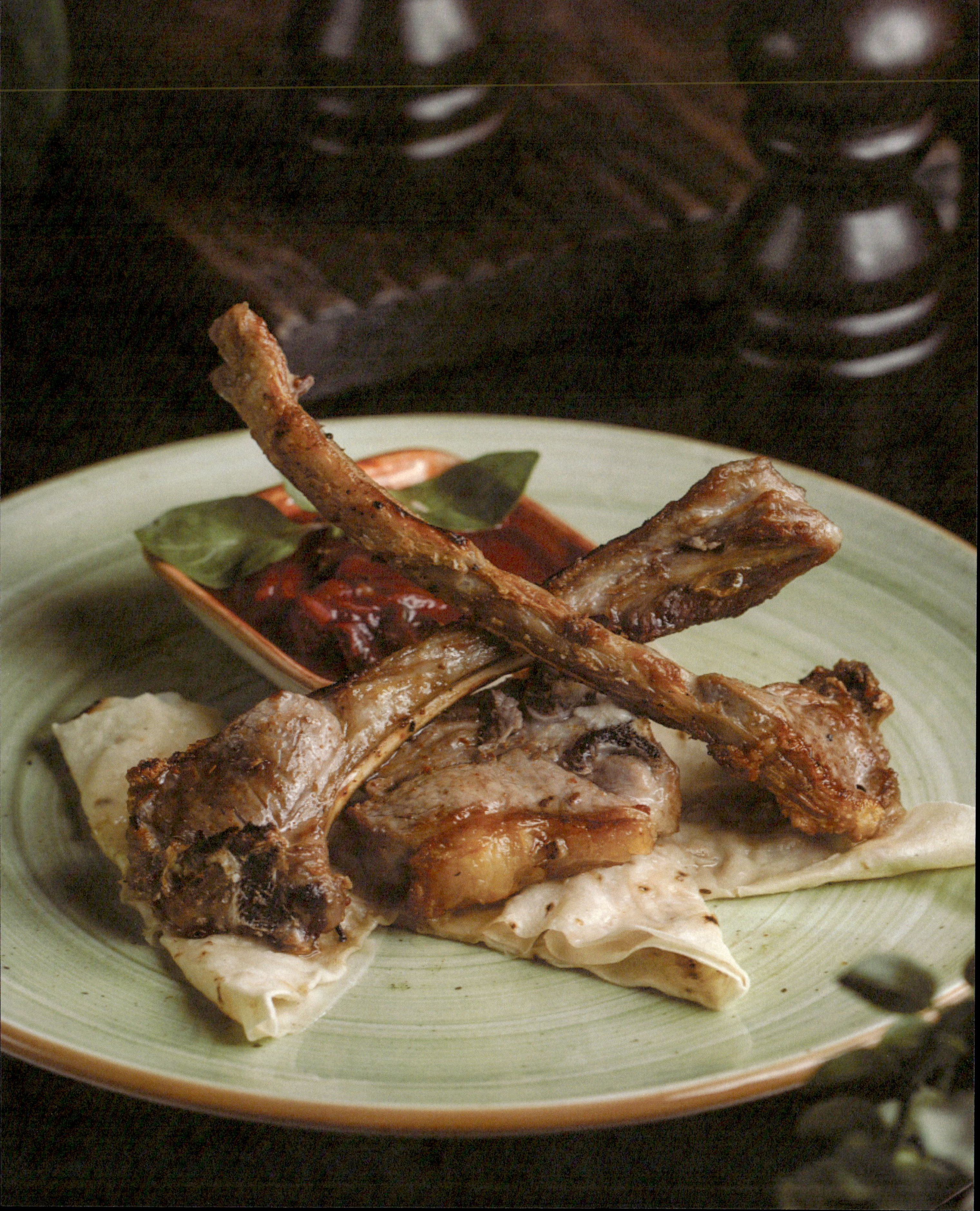

Pear Infused BBQ Lamb Chops

Instructions

1. **Prepare the Marinade:**

   In a Blender, Combine the Diced Pears, Apple Cider Vinegar, Honey, Minced Garlic, Rosemary, Thyme, Olive Oil, Salt, Pepper, Cayenne Pepper, and Smoked Paprika. Blend Until Smooth to Create a Flavorful Marinade.

2. **Marinate the Lamb Chops:**

   Place the Lamb Chops in a Shallow Dish or a Resealable Plastic Bag. Pour the Pear Marinade Over the Lamb, Ensuring Each Chop is Well Coated. Seal the Bag or Cover the Dish and Refrigerate for at Least 2 Hours, or Overnight for Best Results.

3. **Preheat the Grill:**

   Preheat Your Grill to Medium-high Heat. If Using a Charcoal Grill, Ensure the Coals Are Well Lit and Have Settled to a Gray Ash.

4. **Grill the Lamb Chops:**

   Remove the Lamb Chops From the Marinade, Allowing Excess to Drip Off. Place Them on the Grill and Cook for About 4–5 Minutes Per Side, or Until They Reach Your Desired Level of Doneness. Use a Meat Thermometer to Ensure the Internal Temperature Reaches at Least 145°F (63 °C) for Medium-rare.

Ingredients

- 4 Lamb Chops
- 2 Ripe pears, peeled, cored, and diced
- 1/4 cup Apple cider vinegar
- 2 tablespoons Honey
- 3 cloves Garlic, minced
- 1 tablespoon Fresh rosemary, chopped
- 1 tablespoon Fresh thyme, chopped
- 1 tablespoon Olive oil
- Salt and pepper, to taste
- A dash of cayenne pepper (optional)
- 1/2 teaspoon Smoked paprika

5. **Rest and Serve:**

   Once Cooked, Remove the Lamb Chops From the Grill and Let Them REST for 5 Minutes to Allow the Juices to Redistribute. Serve the Chops Hot, Garnished With Fresh Rosemary or Thyme if Desired.

Serving Suggestions:

Pair These Pear-infused Bbq Lamb Chops With a Side of Roasted Vegetables or a Fresh Green Salad for a Delightful Meal That is Both Elegant and Delicious. Enjoy the Sweet, Smoky Flavors That the Pear Marinade Brings to the Dish!

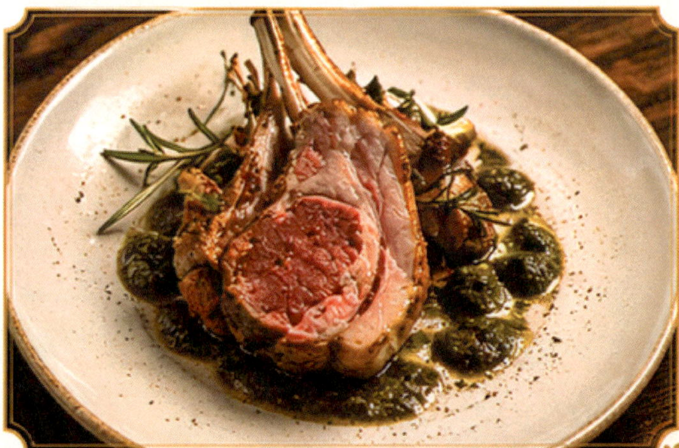

Jerk Chicken Pasta

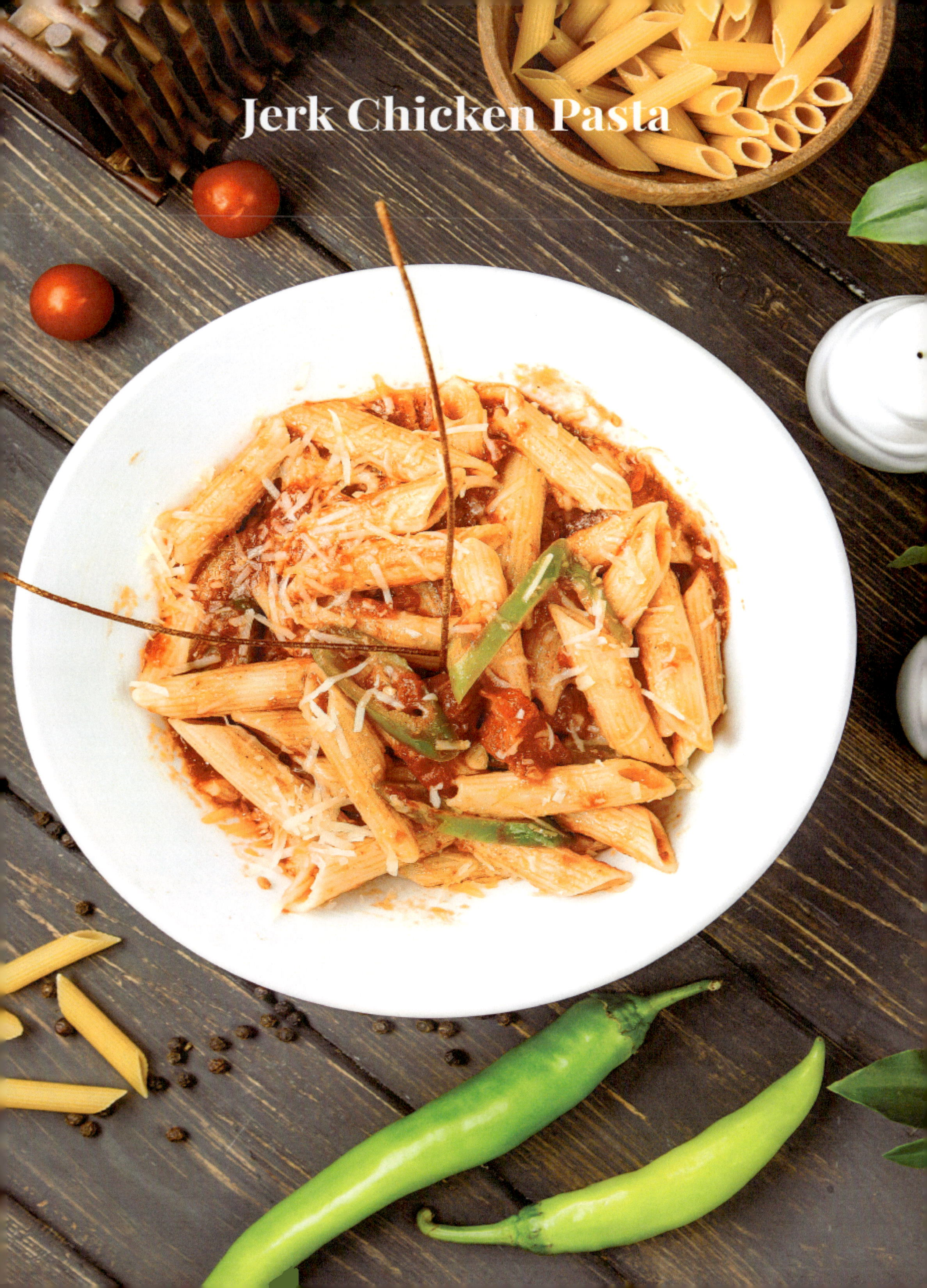

Jerk Chicken Pasta

Jerk Chicken Pasta Recipe

Instructions

1. **Prepare the Chicken:** Rub the Chicken Breasts With Jerk Seasoning, Ensuring They Are Well Coated. Heat Olive Oil in a Large Skillet Over Medium Heat. Cook the Chicken for About 6–7 Minutes on Each Side, or Until Cooked Through and No Longer Pink in the Center. Remove From Skillet and Let REST Before Slicing Into Strips.

2. **Cook the Pasta:** In a Large Pot, Cook the Penne Pasta According to Package Instructions. Drain and Set Aside.

3. **Make the Sauce:** In the Same Skillet Used for the Chicken, Add the Sliced Bell Pepper and Onion. Sauté for 4–5 Minutes Until They Begin to Soften. Add the Minced Garlic and Cook for Another Minute.

4. **Combine Ingredients:** Pour in the Heavy Cream and Chicken Broth, Stirring to Combine. Bring the Mixture to a Simmer, Then Add the Parmesan Cheese, Stirring Until Melted and the Sauce Thickens Slightly. Season With Salt and Pepper to Taste.

5. **Assemble the Dish:** Add the Cooked Pasta and Sliced Chicken to the Sauce. Toss Everything Together Until the Pasta and Chicken Are Well Coated With the Sauce.

Ingredients

- 2 Boneless, Skinless Chicken Breasts
- 2 Tablespoons Jerk Seasoning
- 1 Tablespoon Olive Oil
- 8 Ounces Penne Pasta
- 1 Cup Heavy Cream
- 1 Cup Chicken Broth
- 1/2 Cup Grated Parmesan Cheese
- 1 Red Bell Pepper, Sliced
- 1 Yellow Onion, Sliced
- 2 Cloves Garlic, Minced
- Salt and Pepper, to Taste
- Fresh Parsley, Chopped (for Garnish)

6. **Serve:** Divide the Pasta Among Plates or Bowls. Garnish With Fresh Parsley and Extra Parmesan Cheese if Desired. Enjoy Your Flavorful Jerk Chicken Pasta!

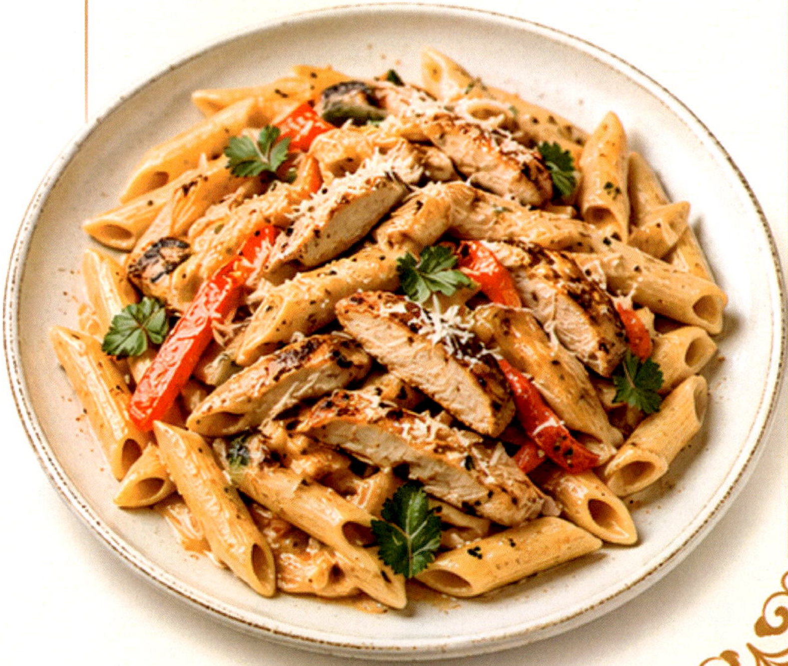

Goldie's Shrimp N Grits

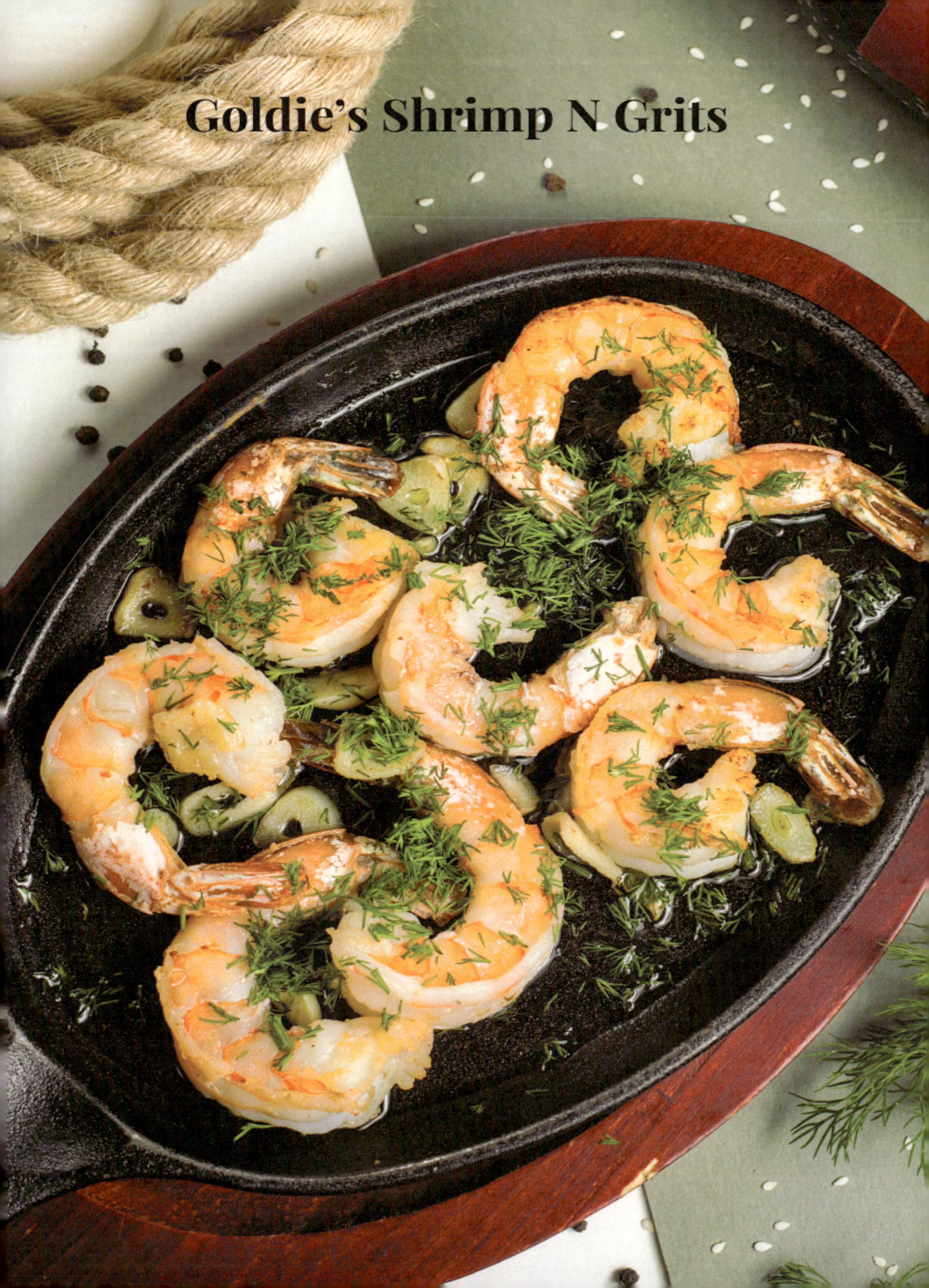

Goldie's Shrimp N Grits

Instructions

1. **Cook the Grits:** In a Medium Saucepan, Bring Water and Milk to a Boil. Gradually Whisk in the Grits, Reducing the Heat to Low. Cook, Stirring Occasionally, Until Thick and Creamy, About 20–25 Minutes. Stir in Butter, Cheddar Cheese, Salt, and Pepper. Keep Warm.

2. **Prepare the Shrimp:** In a Large Skillet, Cook the Bacon Over Medium Heat Until Crispy. Remove Bacon With a Slotted Spoon and Drain on Paper Towels, Leaving the Drippings in the Skillet.

3. **Sauté the Vegetables:** Add Olive Oil to the Skillet With the Bacon Drippings. Sauté the Onion and Bell Pepper Until Soft, About 5 Minutes. Add Garlic and Cook for Another Minute.

4. **Cook the Shrimp:** Add Shrimp to the Skillet, Seasoning With Cajun Seasoning, Cayenne Pepper, Salt, and Pepper. Cook Until Shrimp Are Pink and Opaque, About 3–4 Minutes. Stir in Lemon Juice and Cooked Bacon.

5. **Serve:** Spoon the Creamy Grits Onto Plates or Bowls and Top With the Shrimp Mixture. Garnish With Fresh Parsley and Serve Immediately.

Enjoy Your Southern Style Shrimp and Grits, a Comforting and Flavorful Dish Perfect for Any Occasion!

Ingredients

For the Grits:

- 1 Cup Stone-ground Grits
- 4 Cups Water
- 1 Cup Milk
- 2 Tablespoons Unsalted Butter
- Salt and Pepper to Taste
- 1 Cup Shredded Sharp Cheddar Cheese

For the Shrimp:

- 1 Pound Large Shrimp, Peeled and Deveined
- 4 Slices Bacon, Chopped
- 1 Tablespoon Olive Oil
- 1 Small Onion, Diced
- 1 Bell Pepper, Diced
- 2 Cloves Garlic, Minced
- 1 Teaspoon Cajun Seasoning
- 1/4 Teaspoon Cayenne Pepper (Optional, for Extra Heat)
- Juice of 1 Lemon
- 2 Tablespoons Chopped Fresh Parsley
- Salt and Pepper to Taste

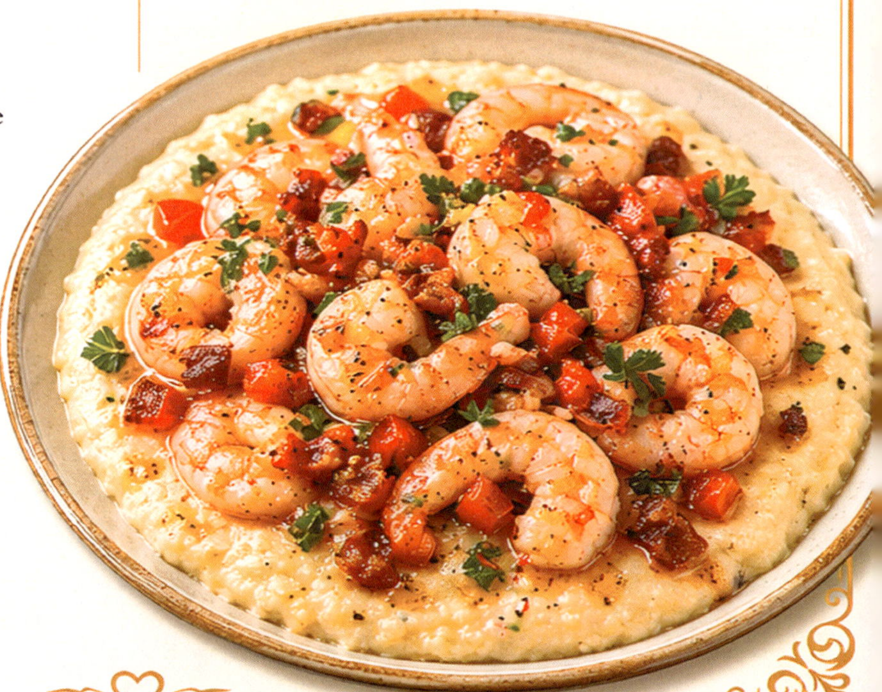

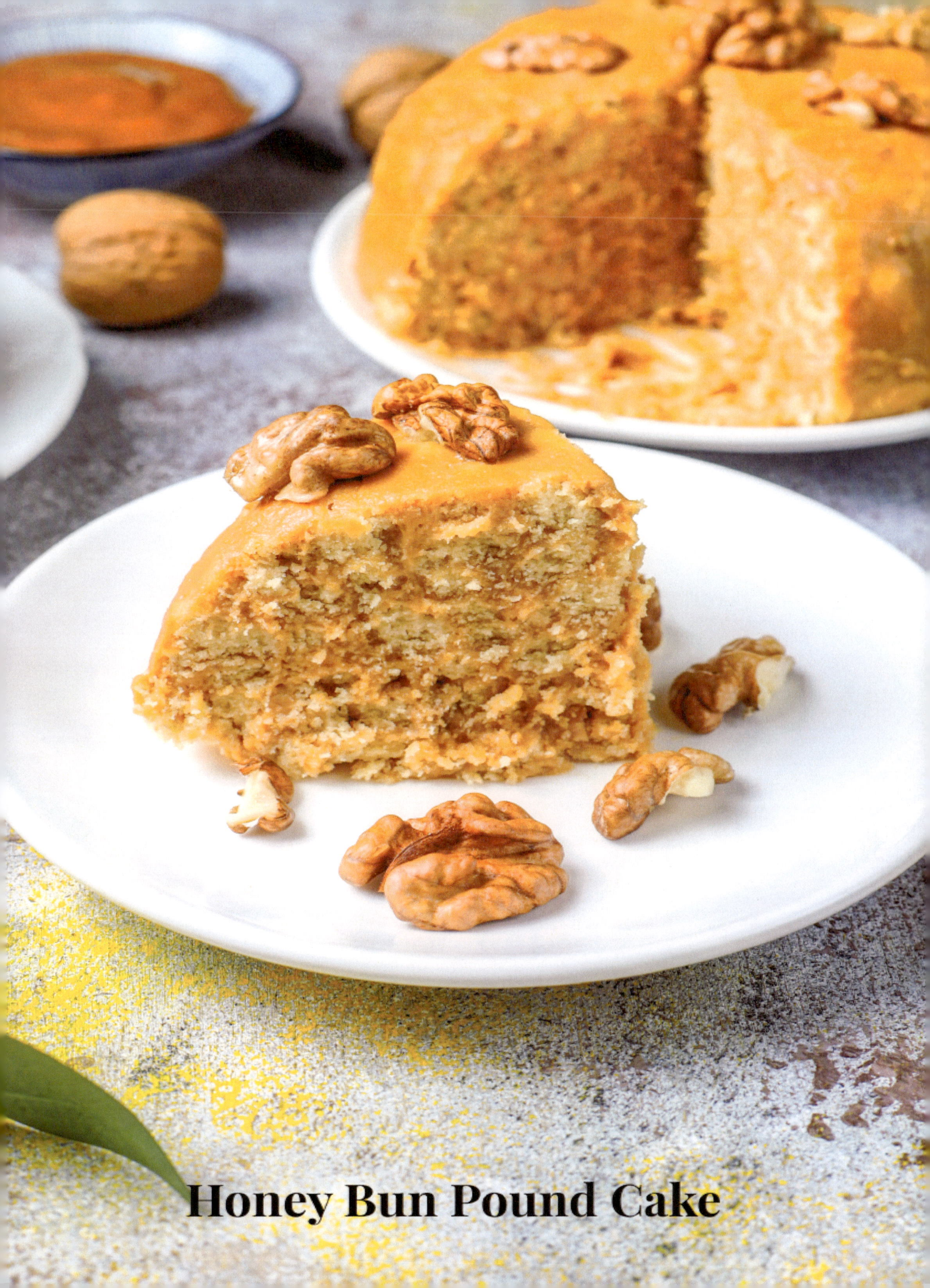

Honey Bun Pound Cake

HONEY BUN POUND CAKE

INSTRUCTIONS

1. PREHEAT OVEN:

- Preheat your oven to 325°F (165°C). Grease and flour a Bundt pan.

2. CREAM BUTTER AND SUGAR:

- In a large mixing bowl, cream the butter and granulated sugar together until light and fluffy. Add the eggs one at a time, beating well after each addition. Stir in the vanilla and almond extracts.

3. MIX DRY INGREDIENTS:

- In a separate bowl, sift together the flour, baking powder, baking soda, and salt.

4. COMBINE INGREDIENTS:

- Gradually add the dry ingredients to the creamed mixture, alternating with the sour cream, starting and ending with the flour mixture. Mix until just combined.

5. SWIRL IN THE GOODNESS:

- In a small bowl, mix the light brown sugar and ground cinnamon. Pour half of the cake batter into the prepared Bundt pan. Drizzle the honey over the batter and sprinkle the cinnamon-sugar mixture evenly. Top with the remaining cake batter.

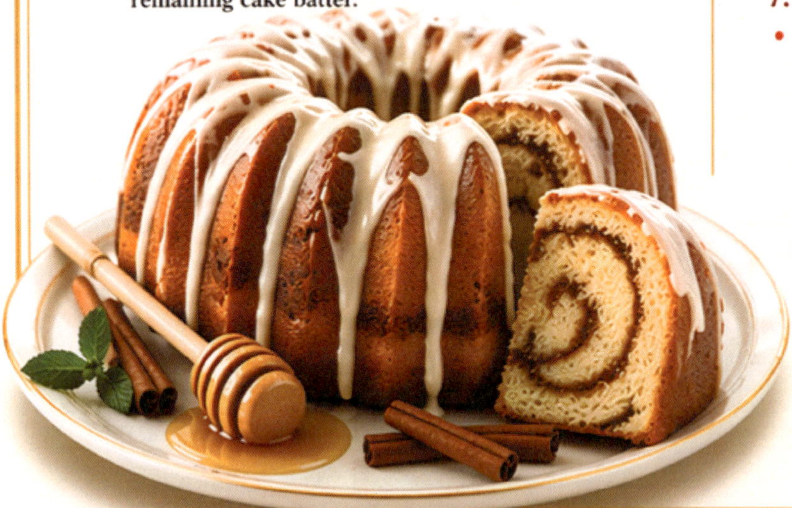

INGREDIENTS

FOR THE CAKE:

- 1 Cup Unsalted Butter, Softened
- 2 Cups Granulated Sugar
- 4 Large Eggs
- 1 Teaspoon Vanilla Extract
- 1 Teaspoon Almond Extract
- 3 Cups All-purpose Flour
- 1 Teaspoon Baking Powder
- 1/2 Teaspoon Baking Soda
- 1/2 Teaspoon Salt
- 1 Cup Sour Cream
- 1/2 Cup Honey
- 1 Cup Light Brown Sugar
- 2 Teaspoons Ground Cinnamon

FOR THE GLAZE:

- 1 Cup Powdered Sugar
- 2 Tablespoons Milk
- 1 Teaspoon Vanilla Extract

6. BAKE TO PERFECTION:

- Bake in the preheated oven for 50–60 minutes, or until a toothpick inserted into the center comes out clean.

7. COOL AND GLAZE:

- Allow the cake to cool in the pan for 10 minutes before inverting it onto a wire rack to cool completely. In a small bowl, whisk together the powdered sugar, milk, and vanilla extract to create the glaze. Drizzle the glaze over the cooled cake.

8. SERVE AND ENJOY:

- Slice and serve this delectable honey cinnamon Bundt cake. Perfect for any occasion!

Salmon Alfredo

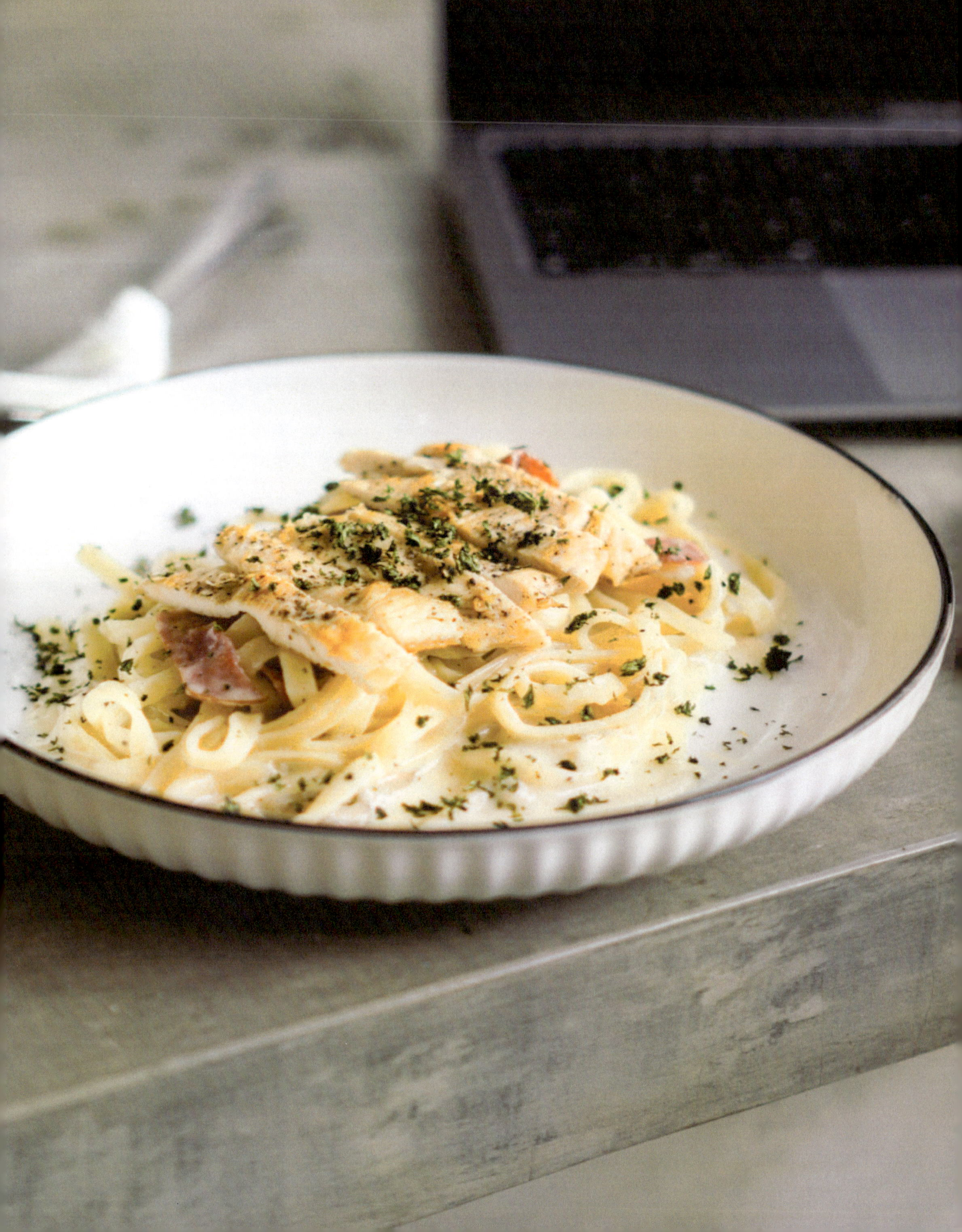

Salmon Alfredo

Instructions

1. Cook the Salmon

- Season the Salmon Fillets With Salt and Pepper.
- In a Large Skillet, Heat the Olive Oil Over Medium-high Heat.
- Add the Salmon Fillets, Skin-side Down, and Cook for About 4–5 Minutes on Each Side, or Until the Salmon is Cooked Through and Flakes Easily With a Fork.
- Remove the Salmon From the Skillet and Set Aside.

2. Cook the Pasta:

- In a Large Pot, Bring Salted Water to a Boil.
- Add the Fettuccine and Cook According to Package Instructions Until Al Dente. Reserve 1/2 Cup of Pasta Water, Then Drain the Pasta.

3. Make the Alfredo Sauce

- In the Same Skillet Used for the Salmon, Melt the Butter Over Medium Heat.
- Add the Minced Garlic and Sauté for About 1 Minute, Until Fragrant.
- Stir in the Heavy Cream and Bring to a Gentle Simmer.
- Gradually Whisk in the Parmesan Cheese Until the Sauce is Smooth and Creamy. If the Sauce is Too Thick, Add a Bit of Reserved Pasta Water to Reach Your Desired Consistency, Season the Sauce With Salt, Pepper, and Nutmeg, if Using.

Ingredients

- 2 Salmon Fillets (About 6 Oz Each)
- Salt and Freshly Ground Black Pepper, to Taste
- 2 Tablespoons Olive Oil
- 8 Oz Fettuccine Pasta
- 2 Tablespoons Unsalted Butter
- 3 Cloves Garlic, Minced
- 1 Cup Heavy Cream
- 1 Cup Freshly Grated Parmesan Cheese
- 1/4 Teaspoon Nutmeg (Optional)
- 2 Tablespoons Fresh Parsley, Chopped (for Garnish)
- Lemon Wedges (Optional, for Serving)

4. Combine and Serve

- Add the Cooked Fettuccine to the Alfredo Sauce, Tossing to Coat the Pasta Evenly.
- Flake the Salmon Into Bite-sized Pieces and Gently Fold It Into the Pasta.
- Garnish With Fresh Parsley and Serve With Lemon Wedges, if Desired.

Enjoy Your Delicious Homemade Salmon Alfredo!

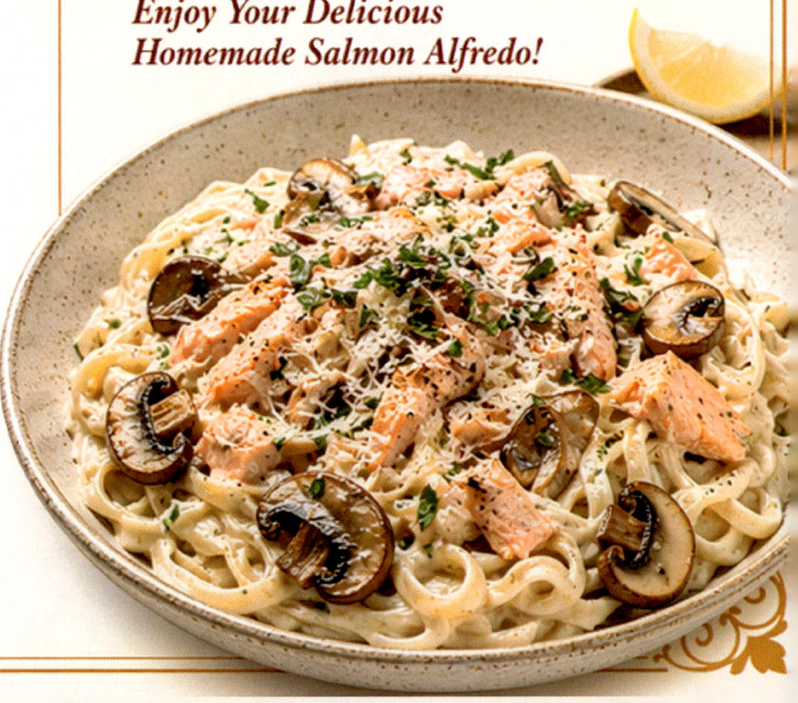

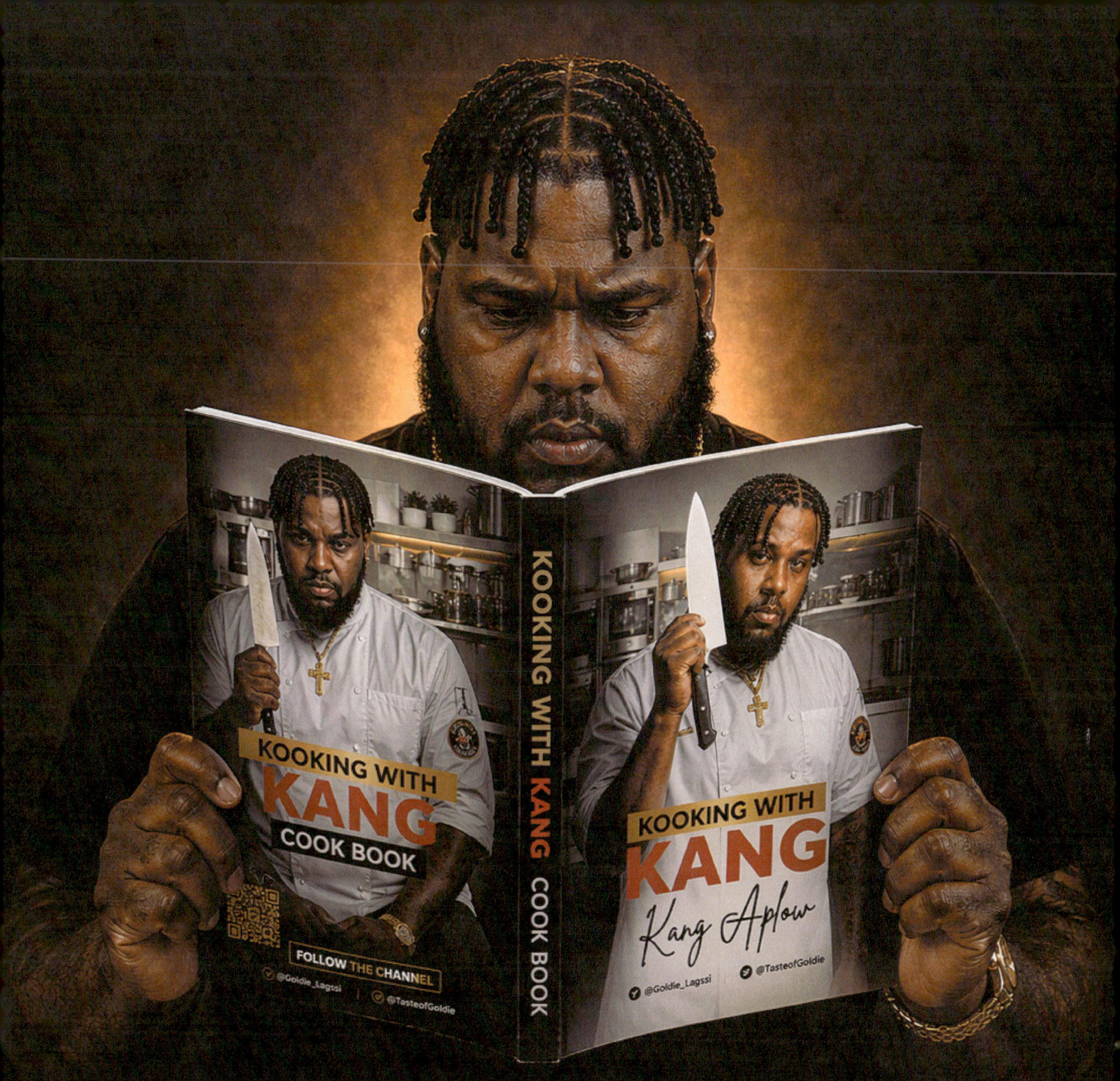

I want to express my deepest gratitude to my wonderful family and friends. Your unwavering support, love, and encouragement have been the secret ingredients behind this cookbook. From taste-testing recipes to sharing cherished memories, you have been my inspiration and joy throughout this journey. Thank you for being by my side and making this dream a reality.

Each page of this cookbook is infused with the laughter and warmth of our shared moments in the kitchen. From the comforting aroma of freshly baked bread to the vibrant colors of a summer salad, every dish tells a story of togetherness and love. I hope these recipes bring as much joy and flavor to your lives as they have to mine. Here's to many more meals shared and memories made around the table. *Bon Appétit!*

www.ingramcontent.com/pod-product-compliance
Lightning Source LLC
Chambersburg PA
CBRC091212220926
51847CB00007B/57

* 9 7 8 1 9 6 8 7 3 2 4 2 4 *